I0413361

Burpees Kick Ass

Burpees Kick Ass

SUCK IT UP AND GET 'EM DONE! THE 10,000 BURPEE CHALLENGE

Sean Davis and Nichole Davis

Copyright © 2016 Sean Davis and Nichole Davis
All rights reserved.

ISBN-13: 9781497533547
ISBN-10: 1497533546
Library of Congress Control Number: 2016910595
CreateSpace Independent Publishing Platform
North Charleston, South Carolina

Contents

Preface

*It is dangerous to be right
in matters on which the established authorities are wrong.*
—VOLTAIRE

The ideas in this book are by no means popular, but they are true. We have seen incredible benefits occur in *everybody* who has completed the challenge. This includes us.

A revolution is taking place. It's not just about an exercise: it's about discovering yourself in a new way. We did the 10,000-Burpee Challenge as an experiment. We did it a couple of times. We had some clients do it. The results were amazing.

Nikki did one hundred burpees a day for one hundred days. Then she kept going—two hundred days, three hundred days. Then she completed the year. The change that took place was shocking!

We made a video to show the world the transformation.* It went viral. People from all over the world related to the 10,000-Burpee Challenge and wanted to do it. It's so simple yet so hard. That is the beauty of this challenge. The benefits go far beyond anything we could imagine. We felt obligated to bring this to the world—meaning *you*!

The transformation that takes place in our boot camps and during the 10,000-Burpee Challenge is more than just physical. We see it all the time. It's like a spark that ignites people's souls—that lifts them and takes them past limitations.

---

* Watch the video of Nikki's transformation here: https://vimeo.com/87858945

They harness that fear, that exhaustion, that pain. They gain strength, hope, and an indomitable spirit. It is incredible to see people's essence, what they are truly made of underneath all the layers. It is sad to see how many people miss out because of fear or ego. We can only guess that this is what differentiates a regular person from a warrior. We are truly honored to be surrounded by such warriors. These people inspire and change the world.

This book is about creating that change in a person in one hundred days. It's more than physical. It's more than wondering if you can lose ten or twenty pounds. It's about igniting a spark that will change your whole life, and this spark comes from handling hard exercise daily.

You might already have that spark and need a new challenge, or you might need to get an edge back in your life. Either way, this book is for you. Here is what you need to do:

1. Read this book.
2. Decide to do the challenge.
3. Join our 10,000-Burpee Challenge Davis Training Boot Camp group here: https://www.facebook.com/groups/10000burpeechallengedavistraining/.
4. Mark your start day on the calendar.
5. Take a picture of yourself after you're finished. Hold up a sign that says "10,000 burpees," your name, and where you are from. E-mail it to davistraining@yahoo.com. We will put your picture on the 10,000-burpee wall on our website!
6. Go forth and kick ass in life with your newfound glory!

Acknowledgments

We are extremely grateful for the support, love, and guidance we have received along our journey. None of this would have been possible without the following:

- God, for guiding us, loving us, and putting this passion into our hearts.
- Bas Rutten and Ross Enamait, for giving us the spark we needed and showing us a new and better way to work out. We hope to give you that same spark.
- Our family, for listening to our endless talks about our business, our workouts, and ourselves.
- Ted Davis and Shirley Davis, who made it possible for our dreams to come true.
- Taylor, Lilly, and Sophia Davis, for being the light of our lives! We love you more than we can ever tell you.
- Our clients and friends who have dared to follow a couple of crazies like us— and found out that maybe we weren't so crazy!

Thank you and welcome to all who become a part of the Davis Training family. Or tribe. Whatever you want to call it. It's an awesome community, and we welcome you! We are truly blessed to do what we do with people like you. And remember, in everything we tell you or inspire you to do, we do it too.

INTRODUCTION

What the Heck Would Possess Someone to Write a Book about Burpees?

An underground revolution, that's what.

We (Nikki and Sean) did 10,000 burpees as a kind of "self-test." It started with Kendell Shewmake and us. We were the owners and leaders of a boot-camp gym. Kendell was one of our members who became an instructor and good friend.

We finished it. One hundred burpees a day for one hundred days straight. The result—we got into amazing shape. But way more important than that, we became mentally tough. We developed a steely resolve that welcomed hard work and sweat with a smile. We forged an inner strength, a sense of pride and self-respect.

We also gained an understanding of how hard completing the challenge is. Its difficulty doesn't lie so much in how hard the one hundred burpees are, although they certainly are tough! The consistency of doing it for one hundred days straight is the real challenge. There are no days off. Even if you don't "feel" like it, you do the burpees. That is what develops the work ethic. Bring your hard hat and bring your lunch pail, because we're going to work!

Along the way of completing the challenge, we ran into all sorts of people who saw what we were doing and amazingly decided to take on the challenge themselves. It's contagious!

Here's a cool story about Kendell and me (Sean). We flew to Oregon to become licensed Bas Rutten kickboxing instructors. We wanted to implement an awesome fight-club program in our gym. All the others there to get licensed were already accomplished martial artists—Krav Maga black belts, that sort of thing. The three-day training was going to be brutal, with ten hours of punching mitts and kicking pads. Oh yeah, and we had our burpees to do. Kendall and I were in the middle of the 10,000-Burpee Challenge.

On day two of the event, Kendell and I were doing twenty burpees during our breaks. We were extremely sore. Everybody was. The instructors asked us why we were doing burpees. We quickly assured them it was because of this silly 10,000-Burpee Challenge we had started and not because the seminar was too easy. They were curious about the challenge and then laughed at us for having to do one hundred burpees *in addition to* our ten hours of kickboxing each day. Well, despite being sore and tired, we stuck to our challenge and did the burpees. No matter what.

The seminar ended, and we all kept in touch. The instructors who put on the seminar decided to incorporate the 10,000-Burpee Challenge with their students. It's contagious!

That's how it works! It's so simple. It's so brutal. It's perfect, really. I cannot tell you how many people we have mentioned the challenge to, and to my surprise, a few weeks later, they tell me they've started the challenge and are two weeks in.

At our boot-camp gym, we trained hundreds of people, and we encouraged our clients to do the challenge. They loved it. People became absolute machines. The ones who finished the challenge gained a confidence in themselves that seeped into every aspect of their lives, and their work capacity went to another level. Scratch that—it went to another freaking *planet*.

And then Nikki took the challenge to a new level. She did the 10,000-Burpee Challenge a second time. She finished one hundred days and then kept going. She did it every day for an entire year—the ultimate testament to consistency. The results were astounding, and we made a video to share the experience. The video about Nikki's transformation ended up being seen by Ross Enamait. The owner of rosstraining.com, he is a legend of a trainer and the ultimate authority in low-tech, high-intensity training. The video inspired Ross to write a blog about consistency, and he shared both the video and Nikki's story.

Well, a quarter million people saw the video on Vimeo and YouTube. The simple concept of the challenge, the consistency that it forces from you, and the toughness of it motivated people to do the challenge. People related to us and were inspired to do the same.

We started getting e-mails and Facebook messages from people all over the world. They were doing the challenge and praising the benefits! From places such as the United States, the United Kingdom, Canada, Australia, and New Zealand, people were sending in photos of themselves as sweaty messes holding up signs that said "10,000-Burpee Challenge completed." The common thread among all the pictures is the look of accomplishment on their faces. These people committed to something hard and saw it through to the end. They changed themselves into stronger, more resilient people one hundred burpees at a time.

We already knew that burpees kicked ass and that this challenge brings people to a whole new level of awesome. But we didn't know how many people were yearning for something like this and that many of them would stick with it and finish the one hundred days.

We should have realized the world is changing in such a way that people crave primal experiences. They want to feel alive! And to be alive is to struggle and sweat and grunt and raise your hand at the end, having endured the battle. Triumphant.

The world is so comfortable and underwhelming now. People want to get that edge back. That's the reason the Tough Mudder and Spartan Race-type obstacle races have become widely popular. We want to experience triumph over obstacles.

We just knew we had to write a book about it. This challenge is life changing. We wrote this book so that we may share with you this gift. This book was written for you. Really.

We sincerely hope you catch the bug and spend the next hundred days obsessing about when you will get your one hundred burpees in.

This isn't a "look-how-great-we-are" book, where we profess to be the greatest exercisers in the world and how easy burpees have become for us. Quite the contrary.

We are, as we finish this book, doing our third 10,000-Burpee Challenge (not counting Nikki's year straight of one hundred burpees). We are humbly reminded daily what it takes to do a hundred burpees a day for one hundred straight days. This shit is hard. Nikki has had surgery and can only do push-ups from her knees. But she is doing them and not giving in to excuses. She is overcoming obstacles by simply refusing to quit and give in. Daily, we are both bent over, our hands on our knees and our chests heaving as we try to catch our breath.

We dread the burpees just like you will for the first few sets every day. After we finish, though, it's a whole different story. We feel as alive as King Leonidas did at the Hot Gates leading his three hundred men. Triumphant. Every single day.

CHAPTER 1

We Used to Be Fat—Did You Know That? Two Stories of Life and Body Transformation

Sean's Story

So, I used to be fat. Want to hear the story? It's pretty crazy how it all came about. In 2009, there was one week when the realization of my fat condition manifested all at once. That week changed everything.

In my midthirties, I took a job as a stockbroker and started eating catered lunches and sitting in my office all day watching two computer screens.

There was always a birthday in the office. When down the hall it was Helen's birthday, I would of course join everyone to sing "Happy Birthday" and eat cake. I could get twenty-five-cent sodas from the soda fridge. Mountain Dew and Pepsi? Yes, please.

Dinnertime? Wholesalers would buy me pizzas I could take home to my family if I just sat and listened to the salespeople talk about their mutual funds for fifteen minutes. For two years, I lived this life, eating like a king and sitting in front of a computer—all day, every day.

I still managed to lift weights about three times a week.

Strike #1

When I was thirty-six years old, I went in for a doctor's appointment because I had a stomachache. The doctor was very alarmed because my weight had ballooned to 270 pounds.

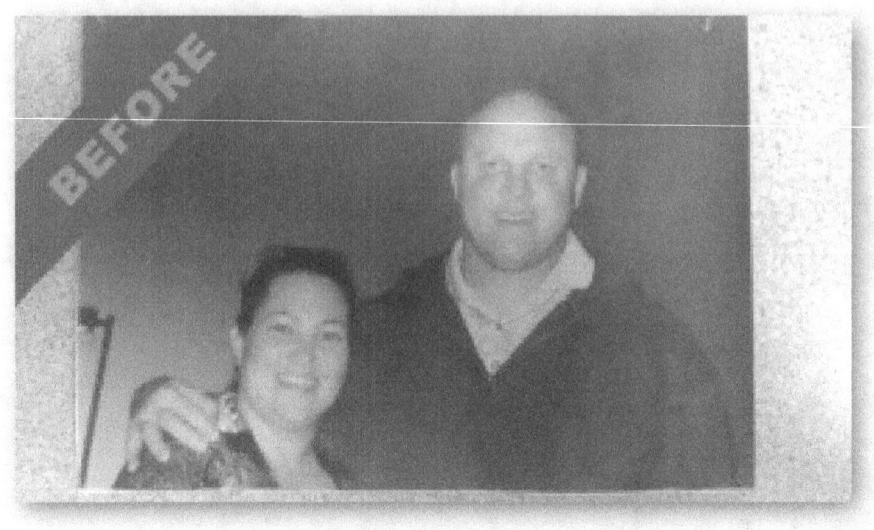

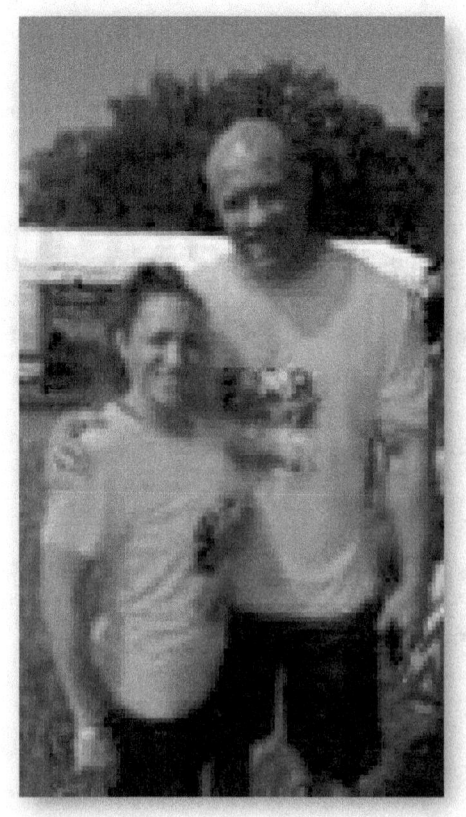

Tests showed that I also had high blood pressure and high cholesterol. The doctor wrote me a prescription for Lipitor, and he was very concerned about my health. When I went home and told my wife, Nikki, she was really upset. I was only thirty-six, and I used to be fairly healthy.

Strike #2

That Wednesday night, I signed up for the church softball team, even though I hadn't played softball in fifteen years. I felt pretty tight before the game, even after I did a few light runs and tried some stretching. I decided that it was only a softball game and couldn't be that physically demanding. I mean, come on, right? It's only softball. I wouldn't be doing any big sprints or anything like that.

Well, I got up to bat, and I hit a grounder to third base. As I ran toward first, the third baseman scooped up the ball and started to throw it to first base. The old athlete in me came alive, dug in, and attempted to outsprint the throw.

Pop! My quad blew. I mean, it blew like a tire that rips off a car, and you see strips of it along the freeway. That was my leg. It was completely torn. Awesome.

Now, let me get this straight: I have high blood pressure and high cholesterol, and I can't run to first base in a softball game without ending up on crutches?

It gets worse.

Strike #3

Two days later, I was sitting at my desk with my two computer screens and talking to a friend on the phone. I had probably just finished eating cake from someone's birthday, but who knows. A few months earlier, I had been out to visit this friend in San Francisco after not seeing him for about ten years. We had run into an actor from a movie set on the streets of San Francisco, and he had taken a picture of the actor and me. Later, my friend e-mailed me the picture. During our conversation, I told him I'd gotten his e-mail. I'll never forget his next words. "It's weird," he said. "You look like you have fifteen pounds of fat on your face."

Excuse me? Are you insane? How about &#%@! you, bro? I thought. But when I looked again at the picture, it was true. I had blubber on my head and face. My belly was big. I looked like a sack of mashed potatoes. My body was like a sack of freaking mashed potatoes.

I hung up the phone and stared at the real me in the picture. Somehow, I hadn't seen it before, as if I had been under a spell that prevented me from seeing my faults. But now, I could see my new fatness in all its glory.

Strike #4

Just when I thought it couldn't possibly get worse, you guessed it—strike four. I know. I know there are only three strikes, but just go with it and let me finish the story.

Fifteen minutes after coming face-to-face with the reality of my ever-expanding waistline, my office phone rang again. John Romero, from my old high school, was calling to inform me that I had been elected to the Hall of Fame for football at my high school. I would be inducted in four months. He asked if I could fly in and accept the honor in person.

I looked at my picture. I had four months to get it together and get in shape. I said, "Yes, I'll be there. And, John…thank you!"

So, in one week, I had been diagnosed with high cholesterol and high blood pressure, had been put on medication, had blown out my quad running to first base, had realized I looked like a bag of mashed potatoes, and had been invited to return to my roots in four months, in all my fatness, to accept my induction into the Hall of Fame for football. That was my week.

I had to get in shape, and I knew that what I had been doing wasn't going to work. I had to get intense; I had to get results quickly. About five years beforehand, when I had joined a kickboxing gym, I'd gotten in super good condition. Fighting shape. We jumped rope and did push-ups, kickboxing, wrestling moves, bear crawls, and so on. When I'd been doing kickboxing, I had abs for the first time ever. But this kickboxing place was hard core; we actually fought each other. I wasn't about to get a black eye or hurt myself anymore.

How could I replicate that intensity? I had some kickboxing workout CDs from Bas Rutten, a mixed-martial artist. The CDs had two-minute and three-minute rounds of simulated sparring. Bas Rutten would announce, "Round one!" and then call out combinations of punches and kicks for you to throw for your choice of rounds. Bas is great! He has a great accent from Holland, and he pushes you and talks you through your workout in a hard-core but sort of funny manner.

An audio program has some cool advantages over traditional DVD programs like P90X or Insanity. I have found that watching a DVD, TV, or computer is distracting to your workout. When you are following a workout that you are watching, you constantly have to train your thoughts and mind on what is happening on the screen. By listening to Rutten's voice shout instructions, you hear the instructions but are able to focus on yourself. Much of my benefit from working out is the presence I get from being focused on a single task. Everything else goes away, and my mind works much better.

For me, those DVD programs keep me distracted, and I don't get the inner solitude that I crave from a workout. The audio workout allowed me to hear the instructions and still focus on kicking ass.

Bas Rutten also has some versions of workouts where he calls out combos, and I would punch accordingly. But then he would say, "Defense!" and I would have to sprawl. Freaking brutal!

Sprawls are where you quickly collapse onto the ground in a push-up position, kick your legs back, and then jump back up to your feet. In football, they are called up-downs. They are similar to burpees, and they are brutal! They disrupt your breathing because you have to drop, stop yourself from hitting the ground, and pop back up. I decided this intense version from "Defense!" was the ticket to my getting in shape.

To start, I did two-minute rounds. Bas would call combos and sprawls for two minutes. I was just shadowboxing, but I could feel all the energy drain from my body. I would do one round for two minutes, lie on the floor gasping, and then do another two-minute round. That was all I could handle—four minutes total. I would work as hard as I could, getting to the point where I felt as if I was drowning from lack of oxygen. For the first week, I did two two-minute rounds every day.

The next week I did three two-minute rounds every day. The week after that, I did four two-minute rounds. I gave 110 percent every minute for every sprawl. Believe me, I needed 110 percent to even get up off the floor each time.

Week by week, I built my way up to doing the whole CD of ten rounds. I was losing weight and feeling fantastic!

One of Bas Rutten's audio workouts is a workout called *The All Around Workout*. It includes shadowboxing, but that is used as a rest interval, called "active rest." The workout is full of thirty-second spurts of push-ups, jump squats, mountain climbers, and ab workouts, and as a "rest," we would shadowbox. The workout is tough and hits your whole body. It is high-intensity interval training. Halfway through the workout, I would have to change my shirt because I had sweat so much. I did this workout every day for forty days straight. The same workout. Every single day.

I channeled my inner athlete—the one that was being inducted into the Hall of Fame. I pushed myself as if I were back on that football field during a fall practice with my buddies. I heard my old coach in my head. I literally returned my mind to the time when I was in the best shape of my life. I went deep into my psyche and felt that same desire, that fire that had propelled me to be a great athlete as a teenager. I lost forty pounds in three months.

I went back to the doctor. My blood pressure was normal, my cholesterol was normal, and my resting heart rate was thirty-six. He freaked out. He told me that Olympic athletes have a resting heart rate in the forties. What was I doing?

I told him the truth. "I am basically flopping down on the ground and getting back up over and over again. I'm doing push-ups and jump squats with no rest, back-to-back, until I feel as if either my heart is going to pop out of my chest or I'm going to puke."

He was blown away. The best part was that I had never even filled my prescription for Lipitor. I did it all with exercise.

I went to that Hall of Fame ceremony and accepted that award. I had found that guy inside me who loved a good competition and who appreciated a challenge! I still had some work to do, but I was on my way! Sean was back, baby!

When I came back from the ceremony, I found I needed some variety in my workouts. I started researching intense exercise. I read *Full Throttle Conditioning* by Ross Enamait, which opened my eyes to a whole new way of working out. Incorporating sprints, burpees, sandbag lifts and carries, jump rope, and sledgehammer, I got in crazy good shape, and I did it all with effort—freaking hard effort. No machines—just my body, my backyard, and a ton of sweat and huffing and puffing.

Six months after I blew my quad running to first base, I even tried out for a semi-pro football team at age thirty-six—and made the team. Think of it: I made a football team consisting of kids just out of college still trying to play ball. It wasn't the NFL by any means, but I was definitely the oldest dude by about ten years.

How did these new workouts work? In my previous workouts, I would never run long distances (more than four hundred meters). But when I ran two miles after six months of training, I got the fastest time ever. This stuff worked! And it wasn't that fake fitness or gym fitness—where you look like a Greek god and can bench-press a couple of plates in the gym but can't run around the block without stopping or jump a fence without pulling a hammy. I could run, jump, lift, carry, pull, and push in all sorts of ways and in any situation. I could do anything! Ready to kick ass and take names! This type of working out worked, and I loved it. I kept trying new things. Every workout was full body and intense with 100 percent effort.

But this book is supposed to be about burpees, so what's with all the talk of these other workouts? Well, we want to tell you how I came to the realization that this low-tech, highly intense style of working out is just the ticket that most people need to get in the best shape of their lives and to get that edge back.

Eight years later, I am still improving. Truthfully, it's what my wife and I have done together from the very beginning. She has done every rep, every burpee, and every crazy, stupid workout with me. I use the word "I" in this book a lot; it really should be "we." We have done this side by side.

We became like workout geniuses. We opened a boot-camp gym in Denver, Colorado, and called it Davis Training Boot Camp. Awesome workouts and exercises just came easily to us after a while. We loved it, lived it, and tried all sorts of things. We came up with different exercises and used the basics in so many different ways. You will see. We have created more than one thousand workouts to get people in shape, and each one is a killer.

We have studied and learned about nutrition, trying to see what works and what doesn't work for us. We have a very clear understanding of what works for people in terms of getting them in badass shape and eating right. We have found the best stuff in terms of exercise and nutrition, tried it ourselves, and then incorporated it into our people's programs.

We have worked with many people and become personal trainers and coaches to more than two hundred people at any one time.

My wife has her own story. She will include it next. Her story is different from mine, and she is amazing. She kicks my butt.

We have introduced this program to many people. Some have bought into it and have given it a real try. Those people have changed their lives. Others have found something else or are still seeking the perfect program. No program is perfect, by the way. Mine isn't. But what it can do for you is awesome, and an awesome workout program can change your life. It changed mine!

Nikki's Story

After giving birth to our third child in August 2008, I was ready to start getting back into shape. Since I had our daughter Lilly in 2002, I had really struggled with my weight. It was an embarrassing and shameful issue for me. I didn't want to be in pictures, and I missed out on playing with my kids at the beach or pool because I didn't want to be seen in a swimsuit. Looking in the mirror and seeing someone I didn't recognize was emotionally exhausting.

Darn it, I was a former college volleyball athlete! I should have been able to run circles around anybody, but here I was—obese. Man, I hate that word. I couldn't—no, wouldn't—admit to myself for a long time that it was what I had become.

In February 2009, Sean found out he was going to be inducted into the football Hall of Fame at his high school. I believe it was in June of 2009 that we were to travel to San Diego for him to be honored. He needed the motivation, and I was definitely ready to start.

We started out doing some rounds of Bas Rutten, a kickboxing workout CD. We could hardly do a minute that first week. We stuck with the Bas Rutten kickboxing workouts exclusively for about six months. Sean then discovered Ross Enamait, and... well, it took off from there.

Listen, ladies, my man lost forty pounds in three months. During that same time, I probably lost four pounds. I am not saying this will happen to you, but it was really annoying and frustrating for me! I'll explain later why it was so hard for me.

Guys, you can skip to the next paragraph because I'm going to talk about breast-feeding. I was still breastfeeding Sophia. I did that with all of our girls for a long time. Unfortunately, I wasn't one of those women who breastfed and the weight fell off. My body is weird. Things usually seem to work the opposite for me, so I struggled on.

When we opened our gym in Colorado, things hadn't changed much for me. Sure, I was stronger and could work out harder, but my weight was not budging. I felt a little ridiculous being a gym owner when I looked the way I did. It was mortifying, but I just kept putting one foot in front of the other. I'd never had a problem losing weight when I was younger. I felt as if something wasn't right, but I didn't know where to start looking.

My nature is to be a really healthy eater. While I was growing up, my family had a garden; we didn't eat a bunch of garbage, and we never really ate fast food. My dad coached us in volleyball and weight training at my high school. My mom competed in bodybuilding, and my sister Ali was a track star. Our family played a lot of sports, and we were always very active.

When I met Sean in 1993, I had never seen anyone who could eat so badly and still look so good. I started getting off track when Sean and I made some not-so-good life choices (something we will share at another time), and junk food became fast and easy. After having kids—and with Sean working fifteen hours a day, six days a week—it became very convenient to eat junk. Over time, my eating habits became more about convenience than about fueling my body. Trying to change my habits was really hard because I was tired all the time.

When we opened Davis Training Boot Camp, we moved from Florida to Colorado. The altitude and cold weather in Colorado was a big shock to my body. I was freezing all the time, and I had developed increasingly debilitating migraines. Although I have had them off and on my entire life, over the last six years or so, they had gotten more frequent and more intense. I was fighting against depression, exhaustion, anxiety, stress, rapid heart rate, and panic attacks. What the heck was happening to me?

Back in the gym, I kept going through the motions, but it was so uncomfortable to be there. How were any of these people going to listen to me? I didn't know what to do, so I just kept putting one foot in front of the other.

We had a miscarriage in May 2010, another one in August 2010, and then in early October I found out I was pregnant again. We lost that baby at around fifteen weeks, in January 2011. I was devastated. I got back into the gym and cried through every workout for months. I needed something to focus on, so I signed Sean and me up for the Colorado Tough Mudder. This is how all our obstacle racing started.

I was so angry, depressed, and exhausted that I struggled through each workout. Others who had signed up to do the Tough Mudder were far ahead of me in their training. I had been training while I was pregnant, but with less intensity than I was training at this point.

This is where the first 10,000-Burpee Challenge was born. We needed a daily challenge to get us ready for the Tough Mudder. The race was going to be intense for sure. Burpees were the epitome of intensity. Especially one hundred of them! We thought, "What if we bathed ourselves head to toe in intensity every day for one hundred days?" What kind of shape could we get into? We were soon going to find out. We decided to do one hundred burpees a day for one hundred days straight. Every day, one hundred burpees. If you miss one day, you owe two hundred the next day. These hundred burpees were in addition to our regular workouts. Extra intensity. Extra work.

I started and completed my first 10,000-Burpee Challenge training for the Tough Mudder, but I ended up getting hurt a month before the race and could not participate. I injured my Achilles tendon and just couldn't run or walk any hills. Here I had put this whole thing together for my gym, and I wasn't even able to compete! It was another blow to add to my already crushed spirit. I spent over a year, from January 2011 to March 2012, depressed, anxious, lost, extremely exhausted, suffering with blinding migraines, and unable to find answers.

Finally, in March 2012, I was diagnosed with the autoimmune disease Hashimoto's thyroiditis, an allergy to gluten, and symptoms of undiagnosed lupus. I also learned that it would be really difficult for me to have any more children—I would need to be on meds, including blood thinners. I am so blessed and grateful for the three healthy, beautiful girls we have. I spent the next nine months researching and changing how I ate. I can't eat like most people. The "no list" includes no gluten, dairy, corn, soy, night-shades foods, pork, or eggs. It has been a very *long* process for me to lose weight. And I still struggle with it every day. Taking medication and eliminating a lot of those foods has helped me drop sixty-five pounds.

I really wanted to do that Tough Mudder! It haunted me that I didn't get to do the first one. Our gym had a team participating for the second year in a row, and no way was I missing this one. I wanted to do it for myself and for my babies that I'd lost. I was worried, though; my autoimmune diagnosis was so new. I had a really hard time with the altitude and was worried because there was a four-thousand-foot elevation change in the race (up a ski mountain). It was also thirteen miles long with twenty-six obstacles.

In all my reading and research, I discovered that people who have my disease are told not to do the kind of workouts I do. I personally don't understand that because I feel they give me more energy and help me deal with the anxiety and depression. Intense workouts have really helped me get to know my body. Still, based on the read-ing, I wavered for a while and finally decided that I would regret it if I didn't try.

Well, I did it! I completed the Tough Mudder and had an amazing time! It was an emotional and spiritually defining moment for me. I was done with limits, expecta-tions, what ifs, others' opinions, and naysayers. I immediately signed up for another obstacle race—the Spartan Race.

It is a daily struggle dealing with my disease; it is a daily struggle dealing with life. I decided to get good at handling struggles daily. I decided to do a second 10,000-Burpee Challenge in April 2013. One hundred burpees a day is a struggle. Bring it on. I had a Spartan Race to conquer!

I just wanted to be more than my illness, more myself. I wanted to find me—that fighter, that phoenix rising out of the ashes of pain, fear, and sorrow. Burpees did this for me. I don't know why, and I don't know how, but I found someone who wanted her life back, who wanted to feel strong. So I kept going with the burpees after I hit ten thousand. Why? Because I loved it! I loved starting my day with something that inspired me to do more. Something that put me in a great mood. Something that got my mind right, opened up my heart, and set my soul on fire. They just became a part of me, so I did a hundred a day for one whole year.

If you want to feel like a badass, do the 10,000-Burpee Challenge. I have seen it transform the body, mind, and soul of those who complete it.

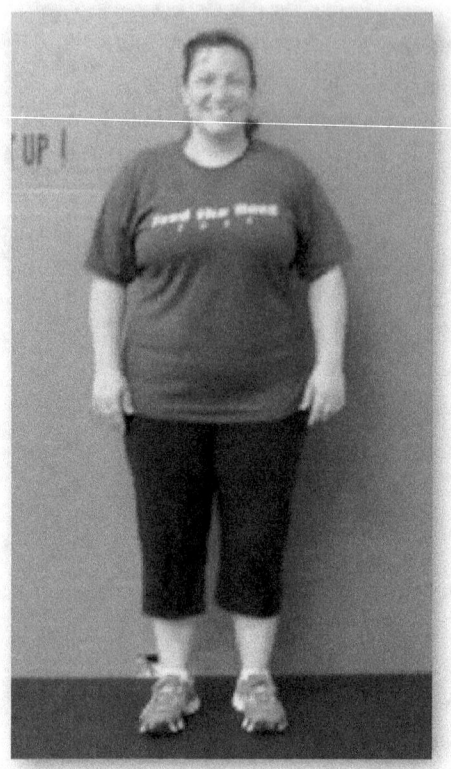

Nikki before

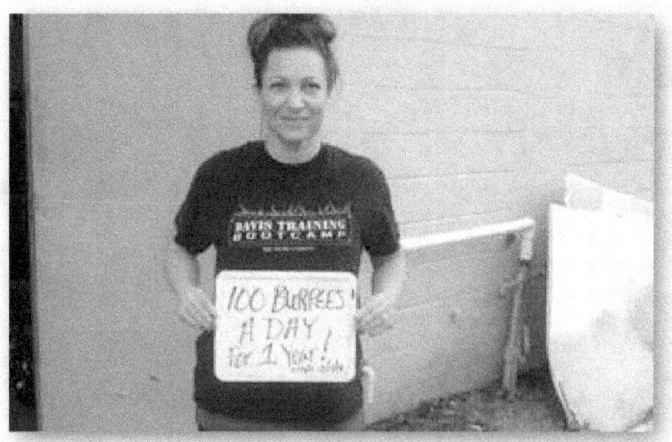

Nikki after a lot of hard work

Don't believe me? That's fine.

Many people won't forge a path on their own until they see that others have done it and realize it's a possibility. I'll tell you a secret. It is much better to forge your own path. Dare to be extraordinary, free of limits, and free of others' opinions. Find you! Know you! Challenge you! Much love to you on your journey. May you find that warrior within and conquer your world.

This book will introduce you to burpees and overall conditioning as a badass way of working out. We will fill you in on the 10,000-Burpee Challenge and get you on your way to becoming a beast of a human being. We will motivate you with awesome mind-set tips. And we will give you more than a hundred totally awesome, adventurous, and brutal workouts—all centered around one hundred burpees. That's right: one hundred different hundred-burpee workouts. But first, let's introduce you to the king of conditioning.

CHAPTER 2

Burpees Are King—They Sit at the Head of the Table and Demand Respect

You enter the gym. You see all the people on the treadmills, ellipticals, and stair mills. They are reading magazines; they are on their phones. Let us state that again. They are "working out," reading a magazine, or surfing the Internet.

You look to the weight room. You see men and women sitting in machines or on benches. They are "lifting." They lift ten reps on the machine and then stroll over to the drinking fountain. They chat with another guy for a few minutes, get back to their machine, lift ten reps, get up and stroll to the drinking fountain (thirsty ten reps, eh?), and chat with the same guy in between sets. Never out of breath, no way, never.

Listen, I (Sean) have managed health clubs for years. I started lifting weights and going to gyms at age thirteen. I am well aware of the culture at health clubs. Compare what you see at health clubs to what you see real-life athletes doing. Compare that to what you see our military doing. Compare that to what you see a boxer doing. They are nothing alike. So, in an attempt to get us in great shape like athletes, US Navy SEALs, and boxers, the health club has failed. It has become comfortable and full of long breaks. It has taken its training principles from nonathletic bodybuilders with large bellies. Seriously. I followed these principles myself until I had my awakening. Before my awakening, I was lifting in the gym, and I developed a giant belly, high cholesterol, and high blood pressure and could not run to first base without tearing my quad muscle. I had to get out of that health-club mind-set. Back to basics. Back to real conditioning. Not sitting in a machine and pulling a lever to flex my muscle but rather using my body as a machine.

I see people all the time get all excited about new machines at a gym. Get on a fake bike or a fake running machine that spins a belt? Does that make sense? Your body is a machine. Move your body rather than moving a machine.

This is a typical health club; there are cardio machines and weights.

Then you see two people in the corner—could be male or female. It doesn't matter. There is no mirror, there is no machine, there is no magazine, there is no phone, and there is no stroll to the water fountain. They have their hands on their knees, and they are bent over and gasping for air. They muster all their will and jump down to the ground in a sprawl. They do a push-up, then they back up and squat, and then they jump into the air. Sweat is dripping onto the floor beneath them. They perform ten of these odd combinations in a row and then put their hands behind their heads, desperately trying to catch their breath and open their lungs. This isn't helping, so they bend over, put their hands on their knees, and gasp for air. They take five big breaths and *bam*. They dive in for another set of ten.

Burpees!

So, here is the truth: the single best exercise you can do is the "burpee." It gives you the most bang for your buck.

Imagine you are on a game show. They put you in a glass box in which money will fall from the ceiling, and you have one minute to grab as many bills as you can. The bills will be in different denominations: one-, five-, ten-, twenty-, and hundred-dollar bills falling down around you. Which bills will you go for? A bunch of one-dollar bills? No, sir! You would go for as many hundred-dollar bills as you could stuff into your pockets.

Why? Because your time is limited! You need as much bang for your buck as you can get. It would take twenty five-dollar bills to equal what you get with a single hundred-dollar bill.

You time is limited, and the burpee is your one-hundred-dollar bill. Go for the big bills! Sure, you can do all sorts of exercises and workout routines. There are thousands of exercises and tens of thousands of workout routines. But the burpee has it all, and you don't need any equipment. You don't need any space, and you can do them in any weather. The burpee develops all five dimensions of fitness: endurance, strength, agility, speed, and flexibility. It also trains a muscle called "digging deep and kicking ass when you are tired." Mental toughness is an asset few have, and you're about to gain it.

Listen—life, games, sports, and careers are won and lost at the very end. The person who can grind it out harder and longer wins. The person who can endure the fatigue and still push through when it's hard—that person I do not want to go up against.

Enduring suffering is an element I include in all my workouts. Always. Get down with pain. Have a seat with pain, share a meal with fatigue, and get to know each other. If you work through some pain, some fatigue, you will grow into a better person.

Now, do not get me wrong—there are many intense exercises out there. But the burpee becomes a mentality that symbolizes the grind. The burpees require guts, balls, whatever you want to call it. They test your mettle.

CHAPTER 3
The 10,000-Burpee Challenge

We did a little experiment in 2010. It was an "experiment" because we didn't know what would happen. We had heard about a hundred-day-burpee challenge, but it started with one burpee the first day, two burpees the second day, three burpees the third day, all the way to one hundred burpees on day one hundred. So you build up to one hundred burpees on the last day. But seriously? One burpee for day one? Nine burpees on day nine?

We wanted to see what it would be like to do one hundred burpees for one hundred days straight. Doing a hundred burpees was such an extremely intense workout for us that we wanted to see what would happen if we exposed ourselves to that kind of extreme repeatedly. So, we did it! We called it the 10,000-Burpee Challenge.

The rules: You have to do one hundred burpees a day, every day. If you miss, you have to make them up. So, if you miss Saturday, then you owe two hundred on Sunday. You skipped Saturday and Sunday? Then it's three hundred burpees on Monday. You must make time—no excuses—and put in the work every dang day.

You also can't do them "ahead." This means that if you do two hundred burpees on Monday, you can't use those extra hundred and just skip Tuesday. You can count the ones in a workout for your own pride, but you can't pay any forward. At the end, you will have completed at least one hundred burpees for one hundred days.

Many people assume you have to do one hundred burpees straight in a row without a break. Not true! We have only done that about ten times, and it was *super* intense. Most people start by doing sets of ten burpees—ten sets of ten burpees and resting in between each set.

One hundred days straight of one hundred burpees! You might be thinking that's crazy. Most people do. But we do not want to be like most people.

Here's what happened to us. We got into the best shape of our lives, and we had already been working out at a very high level. Running? No problem. Three-hour boot camp? No problem. We got into the kind of shape that made us ready for anything.

Let's fast-forward two years. My wife did one hundred burpees a day for a hundred days again, and I did not. It was like an experiment; she was the actual experiment, and I was the control subject. She *added* the burpees to her regular workouts. I just did our regular workouts (and these regular workouts were crazy intense). After about two months, she was crushing me in the workouts. She got such a high work capacity and tolerance for intense exercise that she just blew right by me. At first, she would wait for me, and I would struggle to keep up during our workouts. Then it got pathetic, and I would just wave my hand and say, "Go on without me." The experiment proved one thing to me: adding these burpees to your conditioning program is like squirting lighter fluid on a fire. It ignites your body and mind big time!

We have seen this many times when people in our gym started taking the challenge. It will get you into crazy good shape! Those who keep going with the challenge have a capacity to endure fatigue and do work at a whole different level! Like beasts, they will push harder and longer and kick your butt.

This is what people who have completed the challenge have reported:

- Leaner bodies
- Stronger bodies
- Smaller waist sizes
- Lower blood pressure
- Lower cholesterol
- Unbelievable mental toughness
- Ability to handle any physically tough situation (speed, endurance, or strength)
- A warrior spirit that knows it can do anything
- Confidence that looks fear in the eye and smirks
- A new sense of self that isn't worried about what's in the mirror but about what that person in the mirror can accomplish

In short, they become badass.

This challenge is for you. It's for the common person. It's for the elite athlete who needs more work capacity. Anybody can do it. It just takes steely resolve. Not even much time is required. Heck, you could even break the burpees up into tiny sets of five throughout the day.

Seriously, you don't need anything at all. No gym membership, no DVD, and no personal trainer. You could be in a jail cell with Bubba and complete this thing. All the excuses are gone. We've whittled it down to the bare bones. One freaking exercise. Come on! One hundred burpees. Today, tomorrow, and the next day. What could be simpler? You want us to come over and move your arms and legs for you? This is your life, and we have given you total control.

We have come up with a bunch of workouts all centered around doing a hundred burpees in each workout. Now, if you're already working out and doing intense exercise (which you probably are, as a crazy bastard who bought a book about burpees), we suggest you add the burpees *on top* of your regular workout. So, do your regular workout, and if it includes twenty burpees already, do eighty more during the day. If you do a spin class, then at some point do a hundred burpees too.

It is going to take commitment to start over at zero every day and get your hundred burpees in. Some days will be easier than others. Many days, you won't feel like it. But you do them because you understand that you want to get that edge back. You want that mental toughness that comes from knowing you can do anything. How will you get it? By knowing that you just put yourself through the most intense form of exercise every day. Most people won't ever have the guts to do one hundred burpees even once in their lives. You did it for a hundred days. Just like a recruit in BUD/S SEAL training, no one is forcing you to do this with a gun to your head. You can ring the bell, tap out, and quit anytime you want. But you don't! That's powerful!

You will have an indomitable warrior spirit—a spirit that doesn't quit, that keeps going one inch (or one burpee) at a time.

Don't rely on anyone else for motivation. This is for you. We have done this challenge and have seen many attempt it. Many people give up. Don't put this on anyone else but you! You are the freaking fire-breathing dragon. You are the legend. You are the one who will complete this beast. If you have a partner, that's fine. It helps, but don't let your partner get you negative on your hundred burpees. You are going to grind and finish this!

You have all seen football teams that are flashy and perfect, passing for long yards in their perfectly white jerseys with no grass stains. That's not you, not after the 10,000-Burpee Challenge. You are the team that runs the ball down the other team's throat play after play, physically burying the other team in the dirt. One inch at a time, you pound the other team. Now, you could pass and be flashy if you wanted to, but you have such internal strength and fortitude that you'd just as soon crush your opponent and take their will rather than outrun them.

Burpees! No other exercise strikes as much fear into those that we train. But not you. You are doing the challenge. You see burpees in the workout and smirk. This is where you live, where the only thing that gets you through is the ability to go further into fatigue. When others are backing off, you are just warming up—grunting, spilling a ton of sweat, and accepting oxygen depletion are the only ways to get through. This is where you live!

Is the burpee the "be-all" exercise? We do a lot of different exercises—even in the one hundred workouts in this book—*but* centering your workouts around burpees means centering your workouts around intensity. And intensity works.

How to Do a Burpee

Now, let's get down to the particulars of the burpee. First off, let's just get this out there: you've got to do a push-up in your burpee. There will be those who tell you otherwise. They are weak; you are not. Do a push-up. If you do not do the push-up, close the book, because it's weak sauce. Don't settle for weak sauce.

To do the burpee, go down on your hands and kick your feet out. This will get you in the push-up position. Do a push-up. Then jump both feet back under you. Stand up, jump at least three to six inches off the floor, and reach your arms for the sky. Some people clap overhead, but it's not necessary.

Here are some awesome pictures of the burpee in sequence.

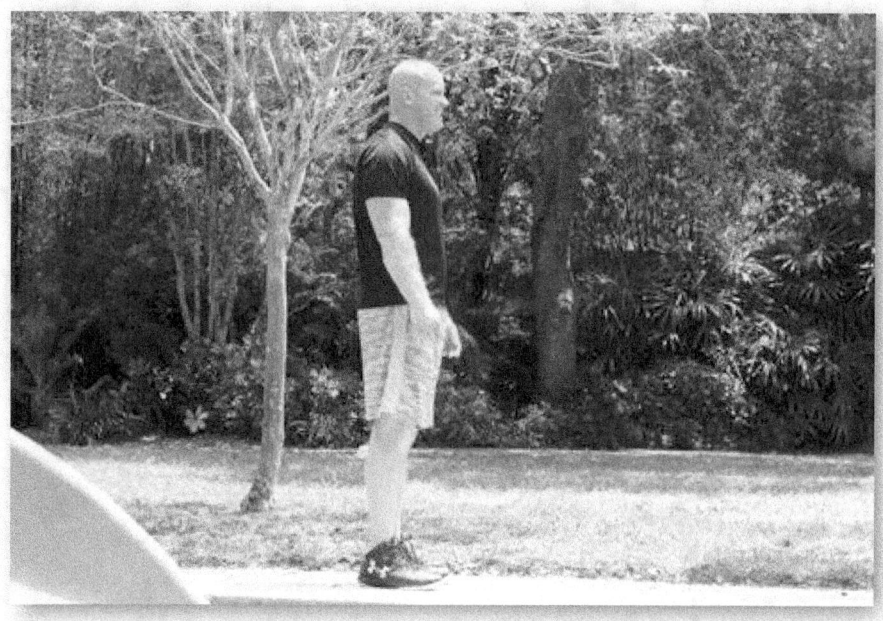

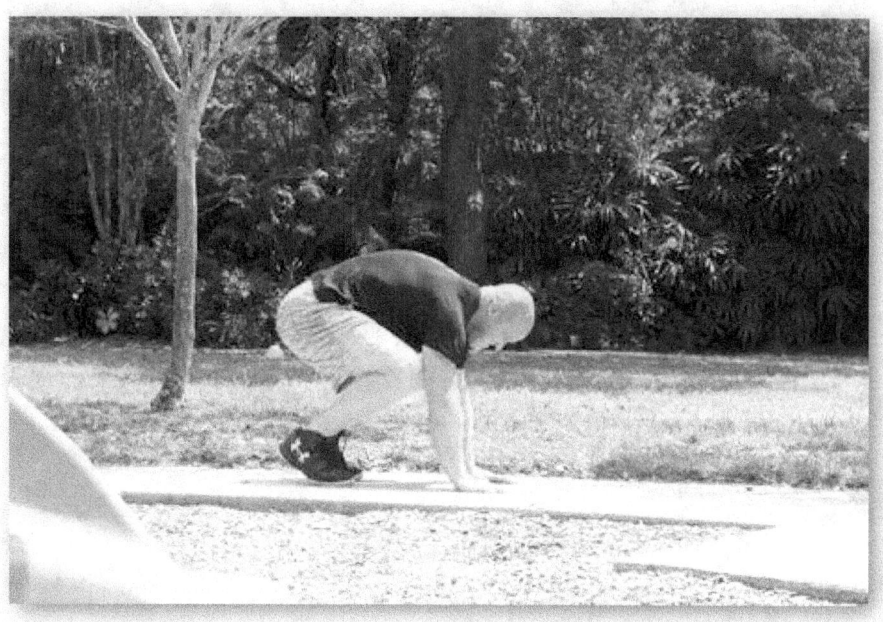

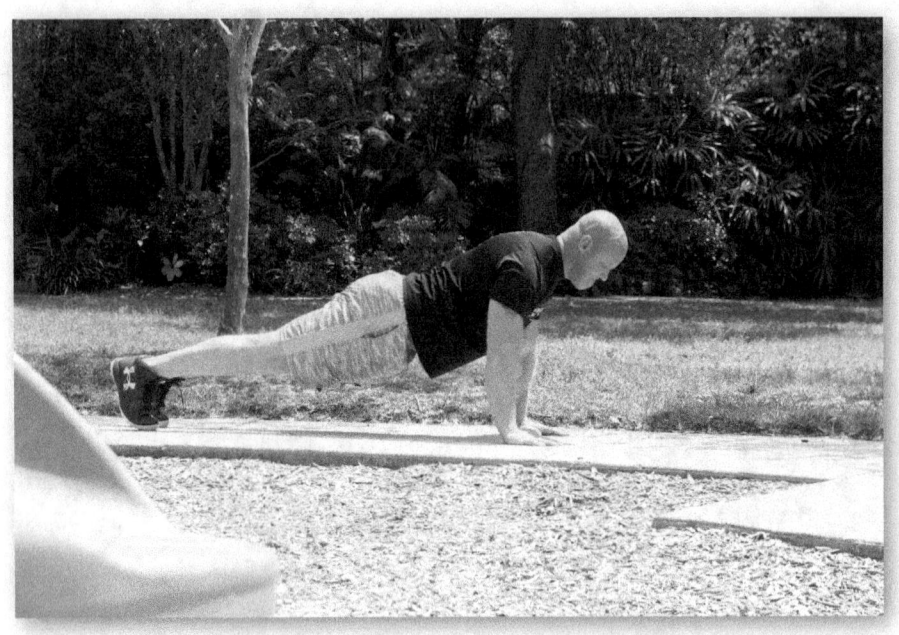

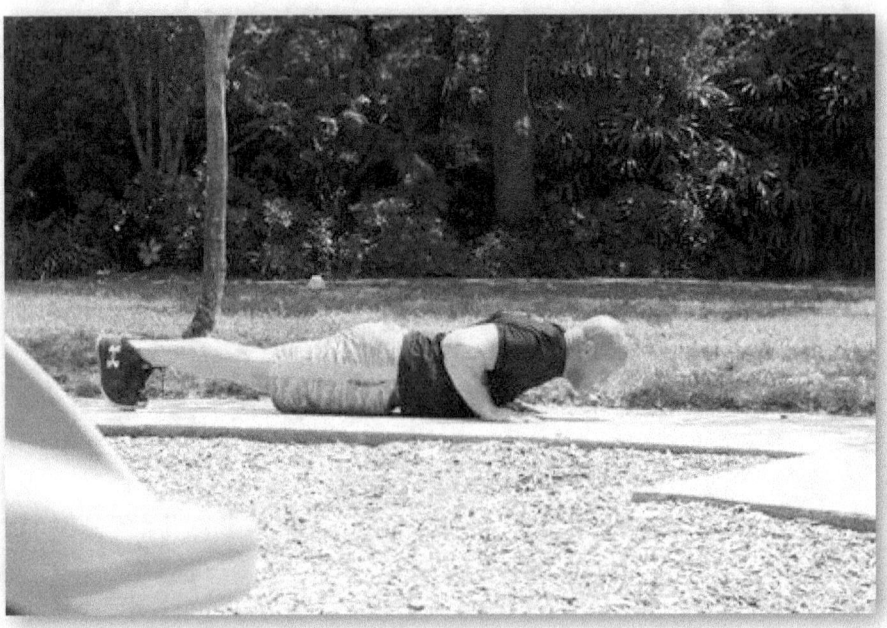

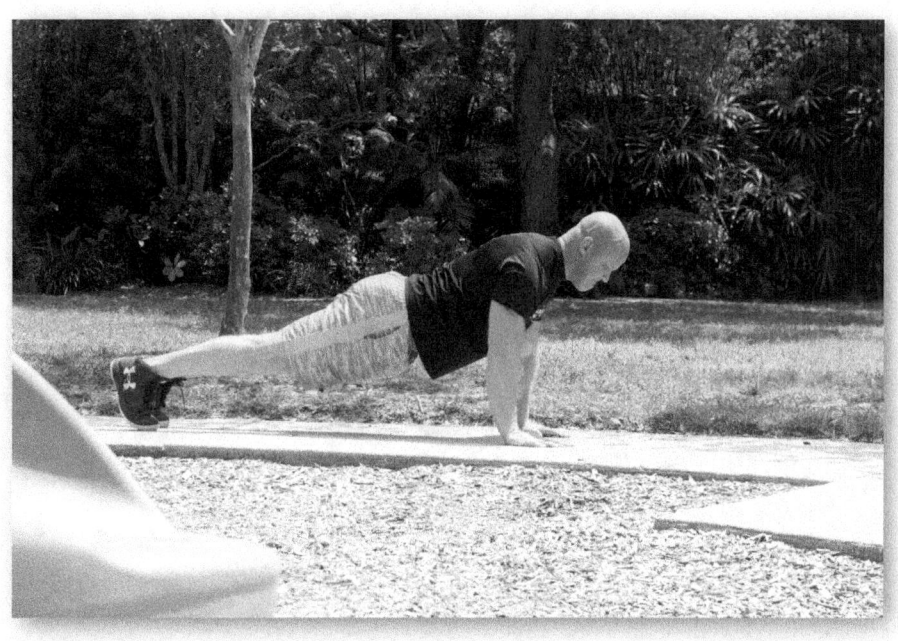

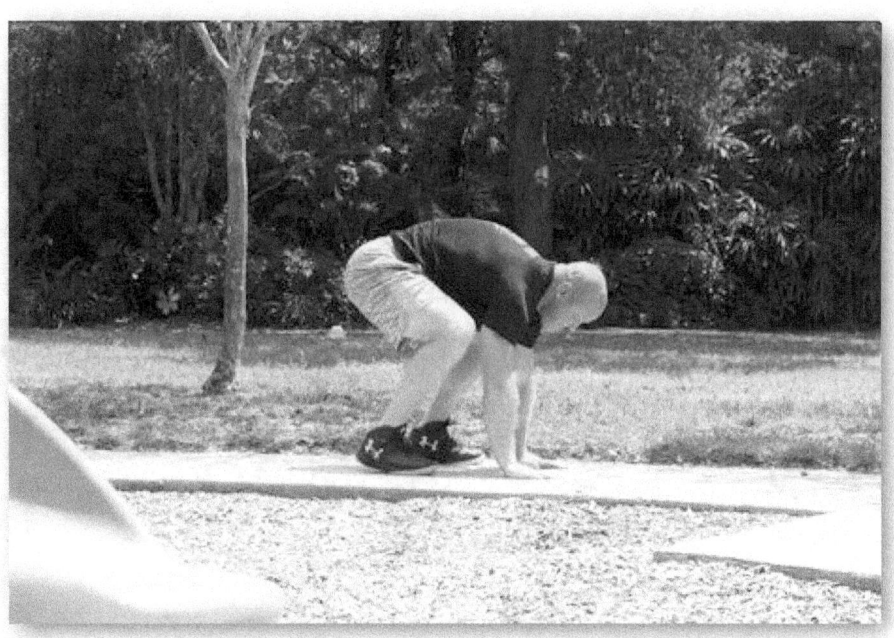

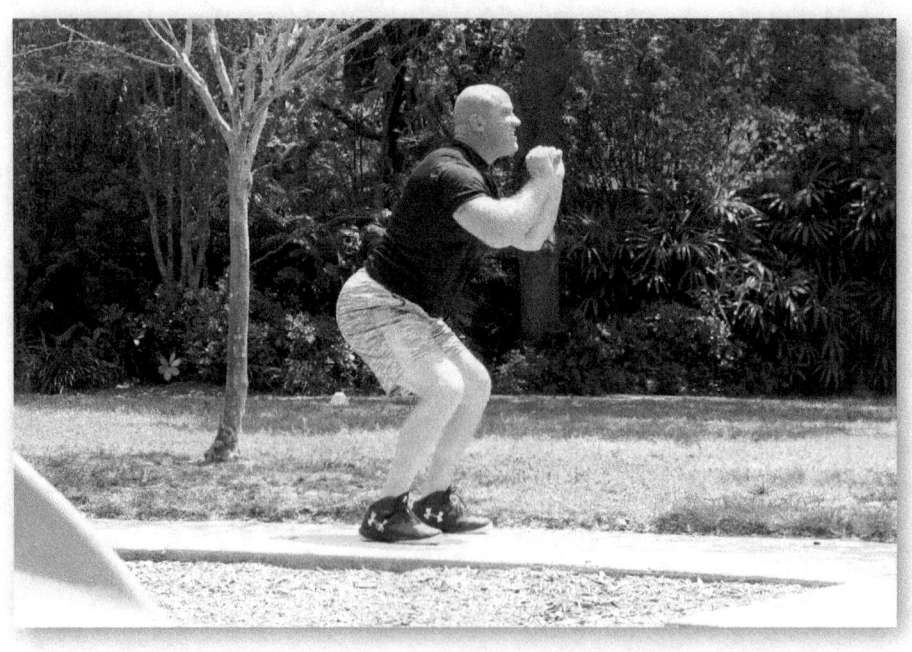

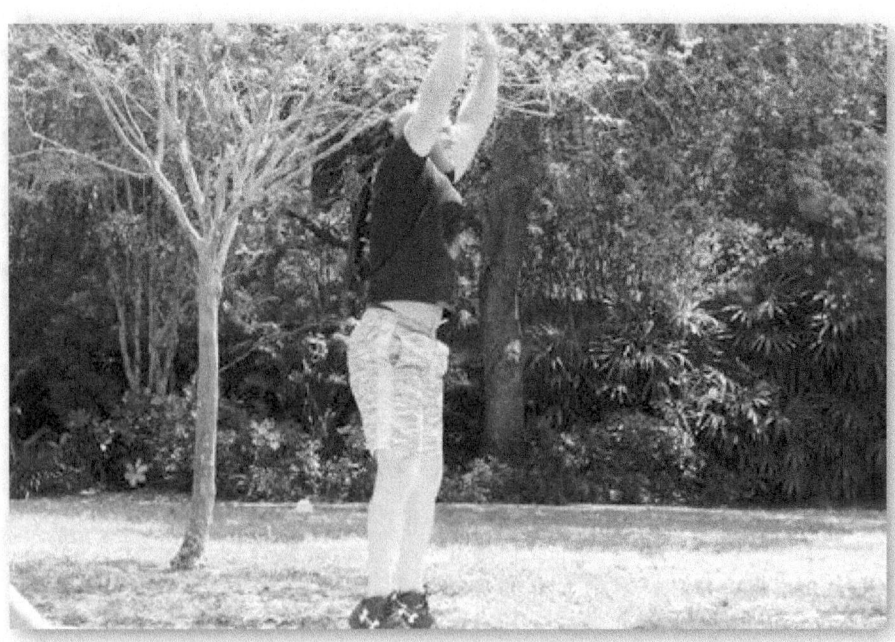

You are performing a sprawl, push-up, squat thrust, squat, and jump all in one exercise. If you have never done burpees before, you'll feel all the energy drain right out of your body with the first ones. That is the magic. That is the intensity you will learn to endure. Enduring that intensity will make all other exercise or less intense activity seem like child's play.

Here's a pet peeve of ours—don't just lie down and get up! We see some people do this in CrossFit. This is not a sport. This is exercise. So, when you do the push-up portion of the burpee, do it right. Get in plank position, lower yourself down into a push-up, and push yourself back up while keeping your body straight and your core tight. Don't just lie down and get up. Have some pride in your burpee. It may take a little longer, but you are benefiting from doing an actual push-up and a plank. You want to strengthen your body, not just flop around.

Another topic we'd like to touch on is adding the burpees to your regular exercise routine. Let's say you're a cyclist and you want better conditioning for your rides. We would not suggest stopping cycling and doing one hundred burpees a day instead. Rather, you should add one hundred burpees a day *in addition to* your normal cycling routine. This will give you the extra mental toughness and the ability to endure fatigue that you are looking for. The same can go for anyone already in a sport or an endeavor. Add the one hundred burpees to your existing program for some insurance that you're going to have an extra gear you can go into when you need it. That's the magic we are after! If you're a boxer, then box *and* do your burpees. If you run, then run *and* do your burpees. If you play basketball, then practice basketball and add in one hundred burpees.

On your days off, burpees keep you in shape. Think about this. Say you wanted to write better, and you decided to spend the next one hundred days writing thirty minutes a day. You would become a better writer, don't you think? That's because you've set up a program with a minimum requirement that forces you to work on your writing every day. Essentially, you would be practicing your writing for one hundred days. Well, in the 10,000-Burpee Challenge, you are practicing your conditioning. One hundred burpees is your minimum requirement.

Some people will not agree with us that the burpee is such a great exercise. That's OK. Those people don't know what we know. They have never led hundreds of people from a nonexistent fitness level to elite fitness. We have.

Naysayers are probably scared. That's because admitting that burpees are king and can have a dramatic effect on your health and fitness means that they should also do burpees. But burpees require the development of mental toughness, and frankly, most people are soft. They like to eat cake. They like air conditioning and the elliptical. They like comfortable, and that's not burpees. No one has ever had the guts to write a book about the burpee. There are over five hundred books about yoga. Plenty of books on squats. This is the first book about the burpee.

This 10,000-Burpee Challenge is a good metaphor for life. Every day, you start over at zero, and you grind to get your hundred burpees. It doesn't matter what happened yesterday; today is a new day. You have been given a new twenty-four hours to get your business done. Doing burpees is your business. Now, get one hundred.

The alarm goes off, and you struggle to get out of bed. You don't want to, but you've got to go out and hunt. Just as the pelican has to show up to snatch a fish, so must you show up for your twenty-four hours. Whether you're sick or feel great, life rewards the survivor—the one who shows up and doesn't quit. Honor your commitment to this challenge. Why is *this* commitment so important to keep? Because you can control this completely.

Not many things in your life are totally under your control. This is. You can control this. You can't control the weather, other people, or the economy. But you *can* find fifteen minutes and do your burpees.

You can.

No time? Total BS! You've got the time, sleepyhead. Here's a trick: get up twenty minutes earlier, or try skipping one episode of "must-watch TV." See, we all make commitments to something. Sean commits to watching five hours of football on Sunday. And he does. We do what we *truly* commit to doing. It's just that many times we commit to crap that doesn't make us better. We commit to Facebook, TV, and sleeping another twenty minutes. What we commit to makes us either better or worse.

Can you imagine if you made a commitment to spend an extra half hour per day on Facebook? In one hundred days, how much benefit would show in your life? I'll answer that for you—zero.

Now, just think. You took my advice, made a decision, and completed one hundred burpees every day for one hundred days. You lost weight around your belly. You got stronger. Your lower back stopped hurting. You were able to run a five K. You tried on clothes and found you have to get a smaller waist size. Your blood pressure is normal. Your cholesterol is normal. You have increased libido. You have the self-assurance that comes from completing a program of intense exercise. You are a better you, mentally and physically.

Which would you choose as your result? Facebook nerd or someone kickin' ass and taking names?

So, now that I've helped you make the right decision, let's get on with this program.

You're welcome.

CHAPTER 4

It's Called Conditioning—Ever Hear of It?

The question: "What muscle does this work?"

Sometimes we get asked this. It usually comes up when somebody is doing a ton of burpees or a full-body exercise designed to get you fatigued.

The answer: You know that muscle where, at the end of a football game, it comes down to one play? Both you and your opponent are tired. He or she is wishing the game would just end already. He or she is tired. You smile a little bit. You've been here before, daily. This is where you live.

You throw off the opponent, overpowering him with your strength. He or she just doesn't have anything left. Unlike you. You burn by him or her and catch the game-winning touchdown. You are hoisted by your teammates onto their shoulders. You are a winner.

That's the muscle this works. The stud muscle.

The coolest thing about getting in crazy good condition is that *anybody* can do it. You don't have to be talented, big or tall, fast, good looking, or athletic. You just have to put in the work. You have to be tough and stick through it a little longer even when you want to quit. Getting into phenomenal condition is available to you and me, and it's impressive no matter who does it.

Ever heard of Tim Tebow? Talentless? Maybe. Winner? Yes. Why? Conditioning. He pushed at the end when everyone else was tired. He outworked everyone, even though some people could argue that he "sucked."

If you've played any sports, then undoubtedly you have played against people who just pushed harder than you did. They went at a faster, more intense pace than you could handle. They just outworked you. It's the ultimate physical advantage in any physical endeavor. Some fighters in the early Ultimate Fighting Championship learned this, and they would just push a crazy pace by getting into extraordinary condition. The opponent would get tired, and that would be it. Now, nearly 100 percent of the fighters are in crazy condition. They have to be, or they lose.

Something exists called the SAID principle. This acronym stands for Specific Adaptation to Imposed Demand. It means that when the body is placed under some form of stress, it starts to make adaptations that will allow the body to get better at withstanding that specific form of stress in the future. For example, Sean needed to pass a firefighter-conditioning test. The test started with three minutes on the stair mill machine wearing a seventy-five-pound weighted vest, and then you had to get off the StairMaster and go through the rest of the course. All the people we talked to said their legs were dead after that, and then they had to try to complete the rest of the course with tired legs. While training for the test, Nikki made Sean use a seventy-five-pound vest and do the step mill for thirty minutes (rather than three). It was brutal! Sean did it three times a week for a month before the test. The point is that we trained specifically to crush the step mill and have fresh legs to finish the rest of the course. Sean's body adapted to doing thirty minutes on the step mill with the weighted vest. When it came time for the test, three minutes of stairs was child's play. That's an example of how to use the SAID principle to become a beast that can't be stopped.

When you do burpees, your cardio and aerobic systems are stressed to the max. Your body needs to use oxygen in a more efficient manner in order to keep up with the demand of the burpees. So, your body adapts, and you become able to push through the fatigue that is inevitable with your hundred burpees. Your body becomes resilient to fatigue and responds to it as if it were a normal situation. No big deal! Just gasping for air! Conditioning is the ultimate advantage in any physical endeavor. If you need to breathe air while doing the activity, then conditioning is king, and burpees are your ticket to the kingdom.

So, if it's so important, why isn't everybody in great condition? Because it is gut-wrenchingly hard work. It's not pretty. No one is cheering you as you are huffing and puffing, carrying a sandbag across the grass at your local park after you just performed twenty burpees. But it is so rewarding. It's life changing, really. You get a renewed mind, body, and spirit. You develop a warrior spirit.

And what's all this talk of sports and winning games? This is a metaphor for life. This conditioning helps you in so many ways. You gain energy throughout the day. Maybe you're usually tired at the end of the day and don't want to make those last few sales calls. Not you, though—you're "conditioned" to push through those last few reps. You pick up that phone and dial a few more numbers.

You feel good about your body, and it's not all about how you look. That's superficial BS. You are leaner and stronger and can do things today that you couldn't last month. You are proud and confident.

Conditioning is king and available to all of us. It requires some work, that's all! Can you do a little work? Or learn to do some work? Then you are on your way, home slice; you are on your way.

Burpees sit at the head of the table when it comes to conditioning. They are hard, mentally and physically. So, let's look at some tips on how to handle that.

CHAPTER 5
Mind-Set

Nothing is good or bad, but thinking makes it so.
—WILLIAM SHAKESPEARE

*A man can only be beaten in two ways: if he
gives up or he dies. Not dead, can't quit.*
—RICHARD "MACK" MACHOWICZ

*Pain is temporary. It may last a minute or an hour or a
day or a year, but eventually it will subside, and something
else will take its place. If I quit, however, it lasts forever.*
—LANCE ARMSTRONG

Your mind is in control of your body. Never forget that. Your attitude, your thoughts, your self-talk, your beliefs—these are what make up your mind-set. And your mind-set is everything. You see, if we did not firmly place the thought in our minds that we *would not stop* doing one hundred burpees a day for one hundred days, we would have stopped. We had to make ourselves believe that we would not stop and then continue to fight the overwhelming urge to just go back to comfortable. Comfortable sucks. Comfortable is fat, and comfortable is underwhelming.

Mind-set is crazy important. We read books about people who push the limits so we can get a look at their mind-set. That's what makes people great. That's what makes them tick. They think differently than others do, and it is a huge advantage. We read about great athletes. We read about US Navy SEALs. We read about great businesspeople who are passionate about what they do. Here are a couple of my favorite attitudes and mind-sets.

Do one extra rep at the end of your workout when it gets hard.

For me (Sean), when I am doing one hundred burpees a day, I am really doing 101 burpees a day. Sometimes it's 110 burpees. I do my hundred burpees (which sometimes sucks). After the hundredth, I do at least one more.

The reason for that extra rep? It's a mental thing. It gives me an edge. I am sneaking in extra work, even on a brutal workout. I always try to live with integrity and hard work. That one extra rep is one of the ways I do that. See, maybe I miscounted my reps. Maybe I did a crappy rep, and this one makes up for it. This helps me keep my integrity. One thing is for sure: I have gotten into the habit of doing more, not less.

Sometimes I do an extra ten reps and tell God that this is my tithe to him for giving me the gifts he has given me. I tell you this not to brag but to inspire, because I generally say nothing when I do this. My workout partners do not know I did an extra rep or ten. I didn't do it for them—I did it for me. It becomes an internal source of strength. It's a mental edge.

You can use this in many different ways—an extra rep or two, an extra set, maybe an extra hundred burpees a day. Do your regular workout, and then run an extra mile. The key word is "extra." If the time runs out on your interval, you finish the set during part of your break.

I used to do this in college while working out with my football buddies when we would lift weights at the gym. I would sneak in extra sets, and it drove them crazy. For instance, we would decide to call it quits after crushing our arms in a workout. While walking out of the gym, I would tell them I was going to get a drink. Instead, I would go to the dumbbells and run the rack. This means I would pick up a weight and do a set until failure, and then I'd drop that weight, grab a weight five pounds lighter, and do a set with that weight. I would run the rack all the way down to the five-pound dumbbells. Extra sets. Extra work. Sneaking it in.

Try it out for yourself. Don't tell anyone, and I promise that you will develop the same edge I get from it.

Not dead. Can't quit.

This mentality is from Richard "Mack" Machowicz, a former US Navy SEAL. You can never quit on life or in life. Let's say you reach the peak of your career. Everything you ever wanted to achieve happens. Then what? Can you hit pause on your life and live in that glorious moment forever? Does life just stop? No, it keeps going. If you are not dead, you can't quit.

We say these four words in our head when we are going through a brutal workout. "Not dead; can't quit."

We say it as much as needed in order to keep those legs churning. Quitting lasts forever. Don't quit.

You can only be beaten in two ways: if you die, or if you quit.

And you ain't quitting.

Be the observer.

The idea of the observer came from Eckhart Tolle's book *The Power of Now*.

When people get out of breath and tired, they tend to panic a little. It feels a little like drowning if you push hard enough and are breathing super hard. Here's what I do. Imagine yourself as a pilot of an airplane. The airplane is your body, and the pilot is your conscious mind. You are the observer, or the pilot inside the airplane. When your body gets stressed from all the exercise, it will start to act differently. You will start breathing really hard, especially at the beginning of the workout. Think of it in terms of the plane going from sitting on the runway to taking off. During takeoff, the engine makes all sorts of sounds and gets really hot and produces a lot of stress on the systems of the plane. You can feel it even while sitting inside the plane. The plane is working harder, and it is very apparent. Your body does the same thing.

So, think of the pilot. The pilot will just observe what the plane is doing, monitor the readings, and steer the machine. The pilot doesn't connect with the way the plane is feeling and want to give the plane a rest because the engine is working so hard. The pilot just controls the machine. He knows that the engine needs to work to get the plane up in the air.

When we get out of breath and start huffing and puffing, we tend to want to relieve that stress by taking a break. But instead, this is what we do. We think to ourselves, *Become the observer.* We start to observe our heavy breathing. We watch what is happening to our body from the cockpit of our conscious mind. It's weird, but it works. Observing it separates you from it. You realize that *you* are not out of breath. *You* are actually just fine. In fact, you are calmly observing yourself gasping for air from seemingly another place. *You are fine.* Your body is showing symptoms of heavy exercise, and that's OK. *You are OK in there.* Your body is tired, but you are just fine!

Now just try to control the breathing. Take big, deep breaths. Like the pilot, just make adjustments and try to enjoy the ride from the comfort of inside the machine. This all sounds crazy metaphysical or whatever, I know. But it works!

Brutal is good.

We make "brutal" a good word. We are looking to reach brutal during a workout. When we feel it, we shout out a battle cry of "Brutal!" And brutal is good. We have gotten to what we seek. Seek after brutal, and embrace it. When the workout gets tough, your legs are dead, and you need to keep going, give a shout: "Brutal!" And then keep going.

"Obstacles are opportunities" is another way of looking at "brutal is good." You want to be challenged. Don't feel sorry for yourself because you are doing a hard workout. Feel sorry for the poor sap that isn't doing a hard workout. That poor sap is going to be dominated by you.

Don't brag. Stay humble. But know…

So, you are going to get through some pretty tough-ass workouts. No doubt about it, these will test your mettle, and you will gain confidence and a sense of pride from doing them. The temptation will be to brag and tell everyone what a badass you are.

Don't do it. Keep that to yourself. Nothing is more impressive than someone who is a lethal fighter or a black belt but then doesn't talk about it. Talking about it takes away from it. It also opens you up for criticism. You don't need anyone else's approval. This stuff is brutal, and you will be a strong human being in so many ways from completing these workouts. You know it, and that's good enough. If others want to try it, that's fine. Then they will really know what you're going through—there will be no doubt. The workout will not lie to them. It will tell them where they stand and show them what they have or don't have. Your job is to be humble and keep on kicking butt and taking names.

Become a leader.

Half the stuff we do is because we lead hundreds of people with our fitness business. We lead by example. For us to quit would mean that we are all talk. Have our people do a workout that we wouldn't or couldn't do? No way. We walk the walk and go through the same pain and emotions as everyone else, showing by our actions what can be accomplished.

We did the hundred burpees for a hundred days first. Then we had other people do it. Your trainer probably won't tell you to do this 10,000-Burpee Challenge because your trainer probably won't do this him- or herself. We stand as an example. We have eyes on us, and they look to us for what's possible. That keeps us going. That keeps us accountable. Like King Leonidas, we suit up in our armor and fight at the front lines with our people. If you are going to die, then we are going to die. We're dying together. There is extreme power in that. Find someone who will die with you!

If you want to have this same pressure and accountability, lead a group or a friend. Become an inspiration to others. You will see that it will make you better.

We always work out at the 6:30 a.m. workout with our group. Now, if we were working out by ourselves, we might just skip a morning or go later. But we have a group of twenty people who will be at the gym at 6:30 a.m. Monday through Friday, whether we feel like it or not. So, we are accountable to those we lead, and we get up *every day* and work out at 6:30 a.m.

So, lead someone!

Dive in.

Doing your burpees or your exercise every day is kind of like showering. Showering is great and makes you feel better when you do it. But there is that very beginning of the shower, when we must get our body wet for the first time. I don't care how warm it is, there is that initial shock when you get your body wet. It also happens when you jump into the pool. Should I jump in fast or wade in slow? You contemplate how to handle the shock.

You go through the same thing with burpees. The first few suck. But the best course of action is to just start. Dive right in. After about twenty or thirty, you are in the groove, ready to kick ass and take names!

At the end, after the workout, you will feel great, just like you feel great after a shower. If you're willing to shower every day so you won't be dirty and stinky, then you can do your burpees every day so you won't be a lump of turd!

CHAPTER 6
The Best Ideas Are Sometimes the Simplest

Simplicity is the ultimate sophistication.
—LEONARDO DA VINCI

For one hundred days, focus on burpees. Focus on intensity. Keep it simple. Like this chapter, simplicity works. Now, let's get to the how.

CHAPTER 7
The Beginner

But what about the beginner?

Don't worry. We feel ya. We've got you covered. Let Sean tell you about his first time doing burpees.

Sean's Introduction to Burpees

The first time I did burpees, I did a hundred of them. I swear. I had no idea what I was about to get into!

I had been doing a routine of push-ups, squats, mountain climbers, and shadow boxing for a few months. I was following along with the Bas Rutten CD workout. I loved it but needed some variety. So, I ordered a book, *Full Throttle Conditioning*, from Ross Enamait. This book came with a DVD of Ross. I got several awesome workouts and a great philosophy from that book, but he kept talking about burpees and referring to a hundred-burpee challenge.

The hundred-burpee challenge is to do a hundred burpees as fast as you can. Well, I read the book and then went to his website and saw people talking about doing a hundred burpees in six to twelve minutes. I thought it couldn't be that hard. I had done "sprawls" before, which are like a burpee except with no push-up or jump. The book and the forums advised that a good way to do them was in ten sets of ten. And they were adamant about the fact that you must do a push-up and a jump.

So, I went into my Florida room (basically an inside back porch), and I started. I went down, did a push-up, jumped my feet back in, and jumped up. One.

Then I did two, then three...by four, all the energy had left my body. I could literally feel the energy leave my upper body as I did the push-ups and then my lower body after I did the jump. Holy smokes! Four burpees? Well, I did ten. Then I bent over, gasping for air. I waited a good minute or two and then did another ten. I felt as if I had sucked on an exhaust pipe! My throat was burning because I was breathing so hard.

To make a long story short, it took about twenty minutes to do forty burpees. That was it. I was done. I quit. I was pissed! And I was sure that no one could do a hundred of those and that all those people in the forum were full of BS! I went into the living room and lay on the couch for about ten minutes, nursing a headache. Then I got up and did ten more.

Rested.

Ten more, and then ten more. Seventy! OK, I can now see the light at the end of the tunnel. I finished the hundred in under an hour. Brutal, beat up, and cheap—but I did it.

I am telling you this story to give you hope and show you that I know what it's like. Everybody starts at different levels. For example, some people can do push-ups without a problem; some people can't do one. We'll cover both below. Some people may be exercising already, but this is a different kind of exercise than what they are used to.

Whatever your story, wherever you come from, you can start doing burpees. Let me give you a starter hundred-day burpee challenge:

Days 1–25:   Twenty-five burpees per day
Days 26–50:   Fifty burpees per day
Days 51–75:   Seventy-five burpees per day
Days 75–100: One hundred burpees per day

Boom! You just committed to a workout program for a hundred days and built up to doing a hundred burpees a day! You are now a beast!

Let's say you can't do a push-up safely from your feet. Instead, you can go to your knees after you shoot your legs back and do a push-up on your knees.

Here is a picture sequence of the bottom portion of a burpee using a knee push-up.

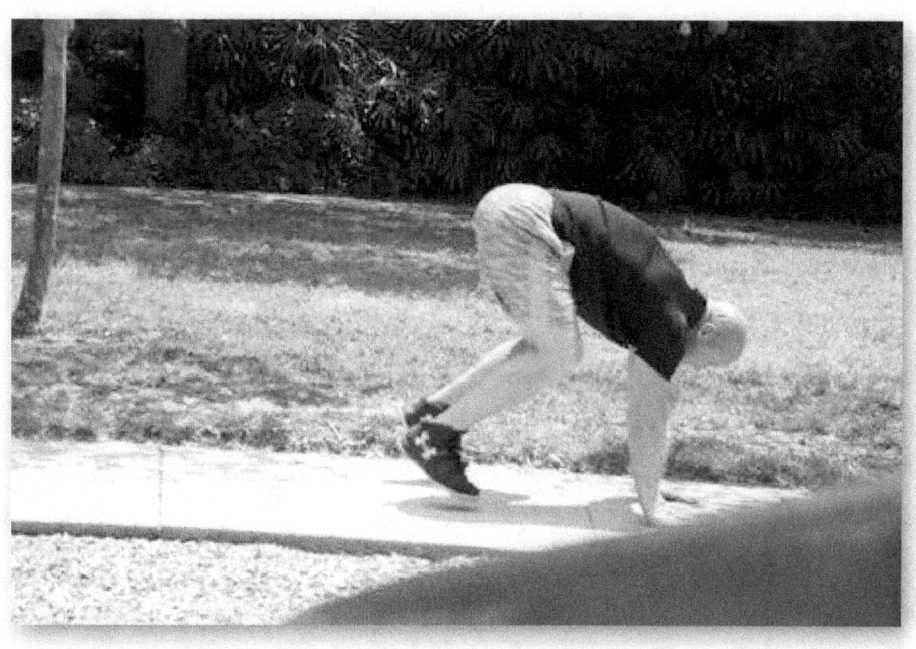

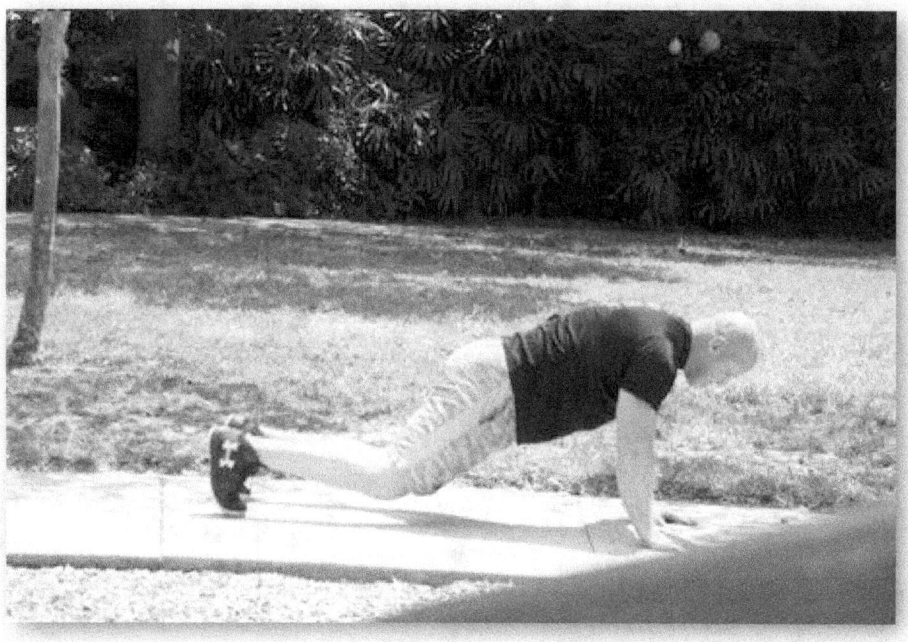

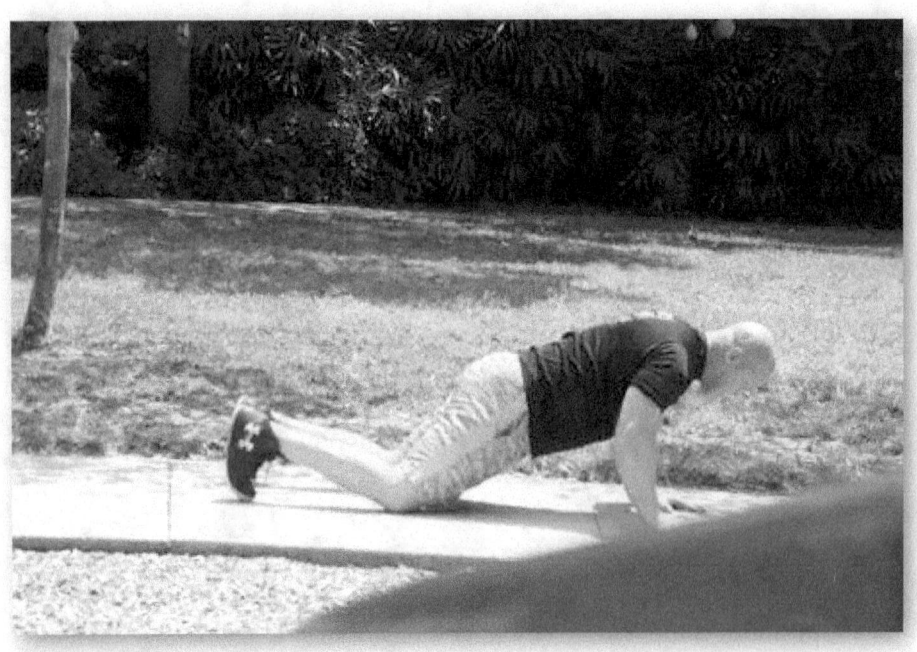

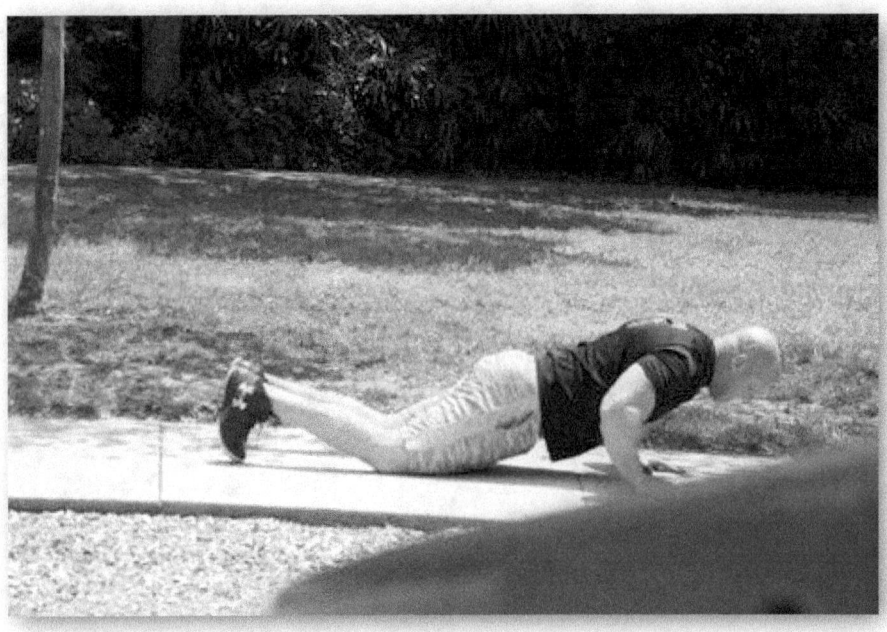

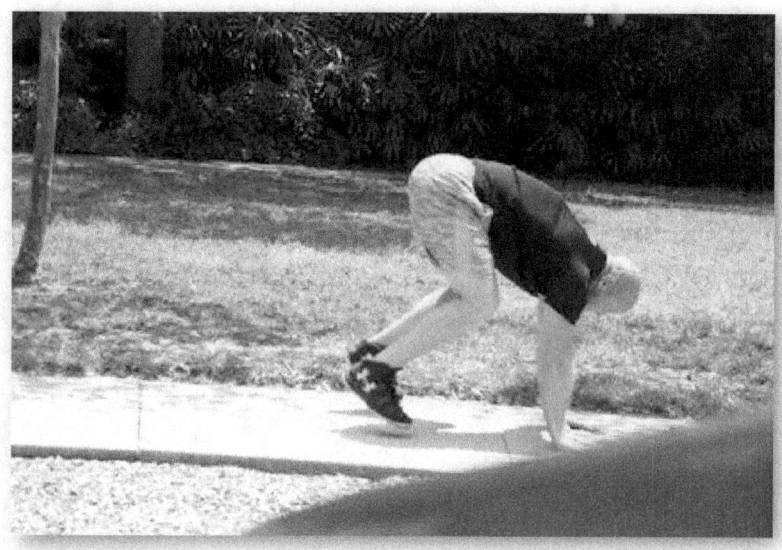

Let's say you can't shoot both legs back at once. From standing, you can put your hands on the ground and then step back one leg at a time into push-up position. (Then do a push-up from your feet or your knees like above.) Then step back one leg at a time. Then stand up and jump.

Here is a picture sequence of stepping back your legs one at a time.

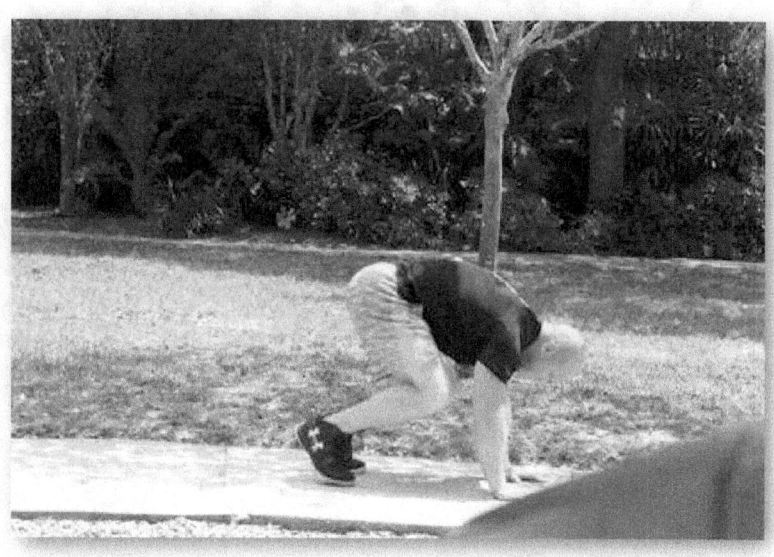

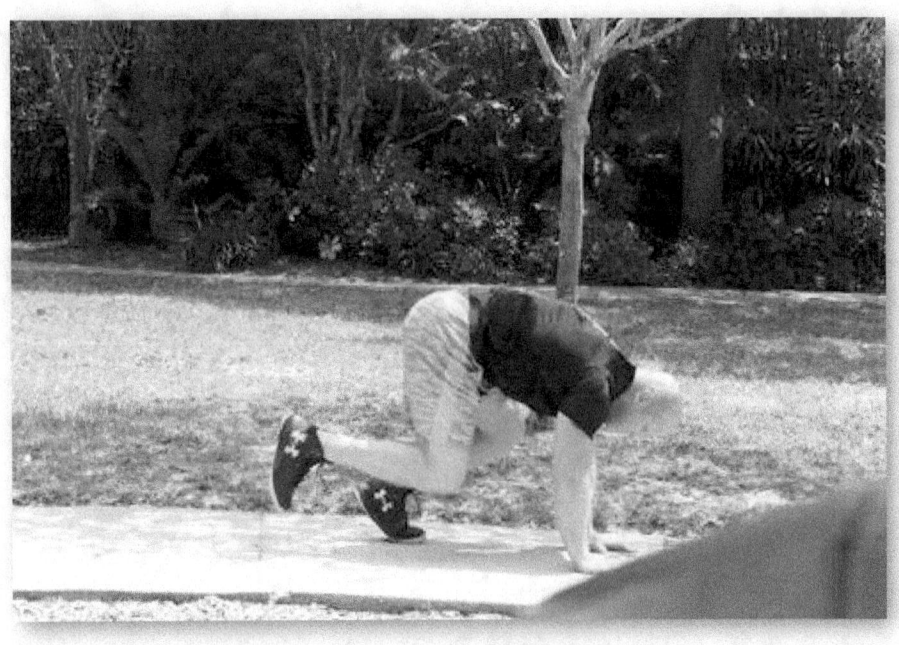

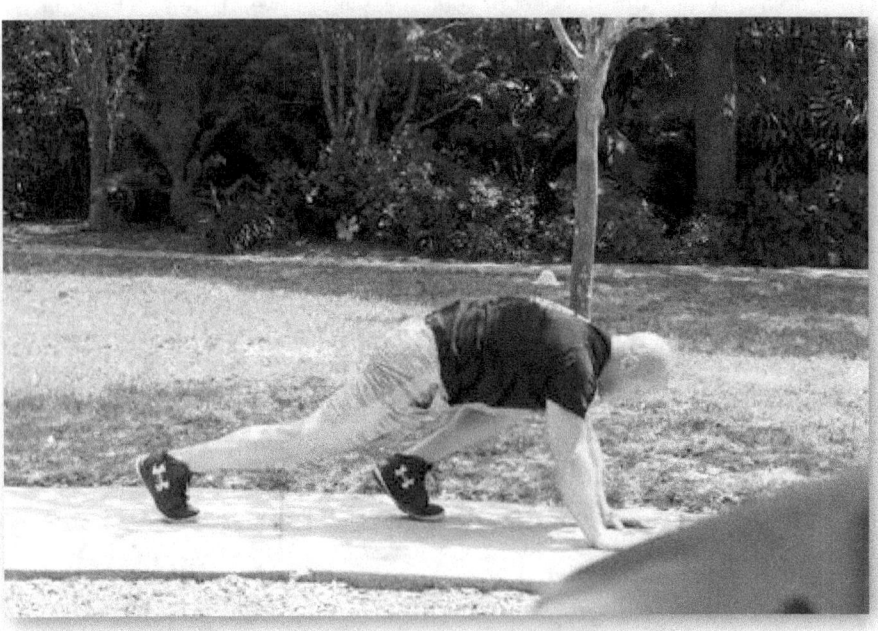

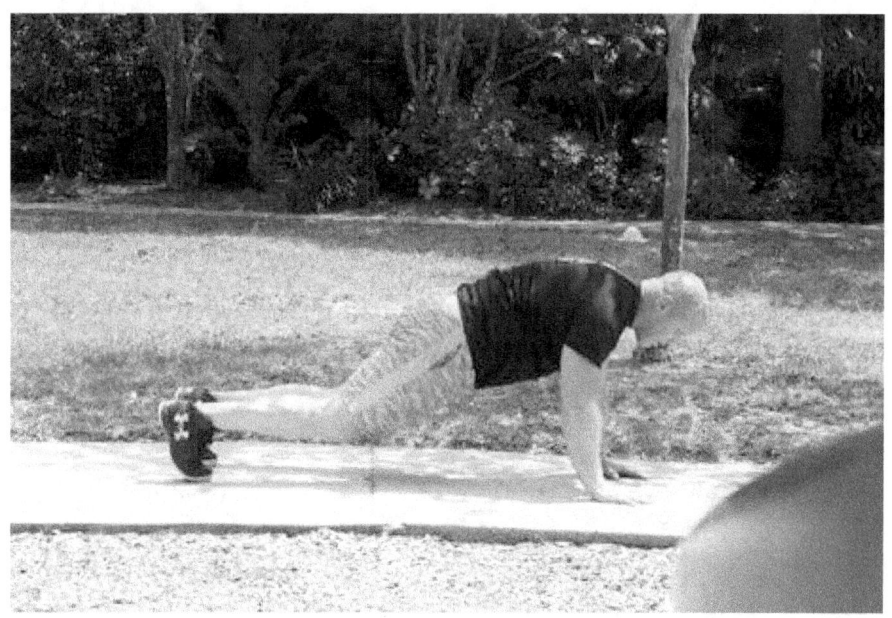

After this sequence, you would do a push-up and then walk your legs back up. One at a time. Then complete the burpee with a jump.

If you can't do push-ups from your knees either, try doing a sprawl with a jump. Essentially, do a burpee without a push-up. (Put your hands down, kick your feet out into push-up position—or step it out—and then jump your legs back in and jump.) You took out the push-up.

I said earlier that taking out the push-up is weak sauce, and it is...if you *can* do a push-up and don't. If you can't do a push-up, you can't do a push-up. That's OK. *But* I want you to do the same number of push-ups using an elevated surface or against a wall as you did burpees. So, if you did twenty-five burpees without a push-up, you should now do twenty-five standing push-ups off a wall or inclined push-ups with your hands on a box or table. The result is that you are working on the push-up and doing a semi burpee. We've all got to start somewhere. You do this work every day, and you will be a beast compared to your former self in a hundred days.

Here is the key. Keep trying to do push-ups. Keep trying to jump both legs back at the same time. Don't get stuck on the wall or your knees or stepping back. Keep focusing on improving those. Now, get to burpeeing!

I heard you guys wanted to see a few workouts.

Drum roll, please...

CHAPTER 8

One Hundred 10,000-Burpee Challenge Workouts

These workouts are in no particular order. Read through them. Pick a few out, and try them. Then try a few more. Figure out what equipment you have available, what space you have (park, home, gym, hotel), the weather, and how much time you have. Also, some of these are just burpees. Some are burpees and full workouts. Figure out what you want each day. Plan your week ahead. Try seven different workouts a week. If you like some of them a lot, keep coming back to those.

Here's a tip that always helps: keep a paper and pen near you, and keep track of your burpees when you take a quick break. Trust me on this. You will get tired, and fatigue makes you forget and gets you confused. You will say to yourself, "Am I on sixty burpees or seventy?" And if you're like me, you don't want to cheat. So, you'll have to go with sixty burpees. If you have a tally of your burpees, it will keep you straight!

I also want to make it clear that these workouts are for variety. You don't have to do all of them or any of them to complete the 10,000-Burpee Challenge. The only thing you need to do to complete the challenge is one hundred burpees a day for one hundred days straight. You can do ten sets of ten burpees every day if you like.

But sometimes you want some spice, some pizazz! That's what these workouts are for!

Here are the workouts:

1. **Twenty Burpees × Five**
2. **Forty, Thirty, Twenty, Ten Running Man**
   Forty burpees, run one hundred yards and back
   Thirty burpees, run

Twenty burpees, run

Ten burpees, run

3. **Fifty Cent**

(Fifty burpees, fifty sit-ups, fifty squats, fifty lunges) × two

4. **The Suck**

(Fifty mountain climbers, three things,* fifteen slams, twenty burpees, ten jump squats, ten jump lunges) × five

*Things = a series of moves with a barbell that makes up one rep. To perform a "thing," take a light barbell (Nikki uses fifty pounds total; Sean uses eighty to one hundred pounds). From the floor, clean it to the rack position. Perform a front squat. Then press it overhead. Then bring it behind your neck and back squat the barbell. Then press it overhead again. Then set the barbell on the floor. That's one rep—clean, front squat, press, back squat, press, and return weight to ground.

5. **Jelly Legs** (warning: this has 120 burpees)

One burpee, fourteen squats

Two burpees, thirteen squats

Three burpees, twelve squats

Four burpees, eleven squats

All the way to fifteen burpees, zero squats

6. **Make It Stop**

Thirty burpees, thirty overhead lunges, frog squats fifty feet, bear crawl back

Twenty-five burpees, twenty-five overhead lunges, frog squats fifty feet, bear crawl back

Twenty burpees, twenty overhead lunges, frog squats fifty feet, bear crawl back

Fifteen burpees, fifteen overhead lunges, frog squat fifty feet, bear crawl back

Ten burpees, ten overhead lunges, frog squat fifty feet, bear crawl back

Good one. If you don't have a plate for the overhead lunges, do regular lunges.

7. **Burpees and Biceps**

(Ten burpees, ten barbell curls) × ten

8. **Not Fully Vested**

Twenty burpees with weighted vest, rest

Thirty burpees, rest

Do this twice for normal days or four times if you need to make up and do two hundred burpees.

9. **Burpees, Box Jumps, and Stuff**

Twenty burpees, ten box jumps, run four hundred meters

Twenty burpees, ten box jumps, fifty barbell squats sixty to eighty pounds

Twenty burpees, ten box jumps, fifteen pull-ups

Twenty burpees, ten box jumps, one hundred mountain climbers

Twenty burpees, ten box jumps, six plank circles

10. **The Flu**

(Ten burpees, prowler sled half suicide, ten burpees) × five

11. **Double Trouble**

Ten burpees, ten dumbbell squat presses every two minutes for twenty minutes

12. **Monkey on Your Back**

Twenty burpees five times, run half a mile with weighted vest

13. **Buck Fifty**

Ten burpees, fifteen slams, five burpees every two minutes for twenty minutes (total of 150 burpees, 150 slams)

14. **Tabata Plus One Hundred Big Bills**

This one is a full workout and requires a little explanation. Perform this workout by doing five rounds of Tabata-style intervals.

Tabata intervals are twenty seconds of exercise followed by ten seconds of rest, done for eight intervals (four minutes).

After each four-minute Tabata interval, you will have three minutes' rest. But the joke is on you! You must complete twenty burpees during that three-minute "rest" period, and *then* you get to rest.

So, the three-minute break starts, and you do your twenty burpees. If you get done with your twenty burpees in one minute, you get two minutes of "real" rest. If it takes you two minutes to do your twenty burpees, you get one minute of rest. It pays to be fast!

Round 1: Tabata medicine ball slams four minutes
Twenty burpees and rest three minutes

Round 2: Tabata weighted squats four minutes
Twenty burpees and rest three minutes

Round 3: Tabata mountain climbers four minutes

	Twenty burpees and rest three minutes
Round 4:	Tabata shoulder press four minutes
	Twenty burpees and rest three minutes
Round 5:	Tabata sit-ups/V-ups (switch back and forth)
	Twenty burpees. Done.

15. Quarters

Twenty-five burpees, twenty-five sit-ups, run half a mile

Twenty-five burpees, twenty-five squats, run half a mile

Twenty-five burpees, twenty-five sit-ups, run half a mile

Twenty-five burpees

16. Twice Is Nice

Ten malligators*

Twenty squat thrusts

Thirty jump lunges

Forty squats

Fifty burpees

Times two

*Malligators are a hybrid between a push-up and a mountain climber. To perform one malligator, do one push-up, and then in push-up position, perform three mountain climbers. It's like this cadence: push-up, three mountain climbers, push-up, three mountain climbers, push-up, three mountain climbers (that's three malligators).

17. Off the Bar

Twenty burpees

Fifty pull-ups (but every time you drop off the bar, do ten burpees until you reach one hundred burpees)

If you need to finish the fifty pull-ups, finish them.

18. Burning Down the House

Twenty burpees

Ten dumbbell squat presses

Ten rows

Long jump fifty feet

Lilly hop* back feet

Five times

*Lilly hop is a traveling exercise. Get in the plank position on your hands and feet, tighten your abs, and "brace" your core. Walk your hands forward. Lilly hops are like a bear crawl, only with the Lilly hop, you stay in the plank and hop your feet forward, trying to keep up with your hands. Walk your hands forward and bounce (hop) your feet forward. If you didn't hop your feet, it would be like walking on your hands in a plank and dragging your feet. So hop! Lilly hops are tough! Our daughter, Lilly, made them up.

19. **Traveling Fool**

> Thirty-three burpees with forward jumps, run one-quarter mile
> Thirty-three burpees with lateral jumps, run one-quarter mile
> Eleven burpees with forward jumps, bear crawl back
> Eleven burpees with forward jumps, bear crawl back
> Twelve burpees with forward jumps, bear crawl back
> Run one-quarter mile

20. **Complex Burpees**

You'll need a light barbell (fifty to seventy pounds for men; twenty-five to thirty-five pounds for women)

> Five clean and press
> Ten front squats
> Ten reverse lunges
> Ten curls
> Twenty burpees
> Five times

Use a light weight. The weight should be light enough to do your weakest exercise without changing the weights. The idea is to do all four exercises for a number of reps without taking a break. Rest after you complete the complex before the burpees. It is brutal—strength *and* cardio!

21. **At Least It Gets Easier**

This will be two hundred burpees (if you missed a day)

> Sixty burpees, rest one or two minutes
> Fifty burpees, rest one or two minutes
> Forty burpees, rest one or two minutes
> Thirty burpees, rest one or two minutes
> Twenty burpees. Done.

22. **Crushed**

> One hundred jump rope
> Ten rows
> Ten burpees

Ten slams

Ten donkey kicks

Ten times

This one is *killer* and lasts forty-five minutes or so.

23. **Every Two Minutes**

(Twenty burpees every two minutes) × five

Rest for the remainder of the two minutes.

24. **Summer School**

If you owe two hundred.

(Fifty burpees, sprint one hundred yards down and back) × four

We would do twenty burpees, rest a little, and then do five burpees and take five big breaths until we hit fifty. It was great!

25. **Two-Mile Century Club**

Twenty-five burpees, run half a mile

Twenty-five burpees, run half a mile

Twenty-five burpees, run half a mile

Twenty-five burpees, run half a mile

Burpees and running always make a great combo. You can't go wrong!

26. **Sprint Slurpees! (Slams and Burpees)**

(Twenty-five burpees, sprint one hundred yards down and back, twenty-five slams) × four

27. **Conan the Barbarian**

Forty burpees, weighted run for about a quarter mile, one hundred jump rope, ten DB lunges

Thirty burpees, weighted run for about a quarter mile, one hundred jump rope, ten DB lunges

Twenty burpees, weighted run for about a quarter mile, one hundred jump rope, ten DB lunges

Ten burpees, weighted run for about one-quarter mile, one hundred jump rope, ten DB lunges

28. **Variety Pack**

Ten burpees

Ten SDBs

Ten box-jump burpees

Ten burpees forward jumps

Ten burpees side-to-side jumps

Ten around-the-world burpees
Ten burpee pull-ups
Ten walking mountain-climber burpees
Ten burpee dumbbells
Ten burpees

29. **Things**

(Five things,* ten burpees) ten times

*Things = a series of moves with a barbell that makes up one rep. To perform a "thing," take a light barbell (Nikki uses fifty pounds total; Sean uses eighty to one hundred pounds). From the floor, clean it to the rack position. Perform a front squat. Then press it overhead. Then bring it behind your neck and back squat the barbell. Then press it overhead again. Then set the barbell on the floor. That's one rep—clean, front squat, press, back squat, press, return weight to ground.

30. **Rocky Balboa**

(Ten burpees, ten run fifty feet, ten sit-ups) × ten

31. **Smoked**

(Ten burpees, ten knee tucks) × ten

32. **Bas Rutten**

(Fifty burpees and a two-minute boxing round†) × four = two hundred burpees

33. **Tyson**

(Twenty burpees, twenty barbell squats (sixty to one hundred pounds), a two-minute boxing round) × five

34. **Rough Stuff**

Twenty-five weighted burpees
Twenty-five burpee pull-ups
Twenty-five burpees
Twenty-five tire-flip burpees

35. **Back and Burpees**

Three sets of max pull-ups, each set followed by ten burpees
Three sets T-bar row with ten reps, each set followed by ten burpees
Four sets low cable row, each set followed by ten burpees

---

† If you are not experienced in boxing, just fake punch the air and bounce around on your feet for two minutes.

36. Manly

>Twenty burpees
>
>Max reps 135-pound bench (or whatever weight works for you)
>
>Run four hundred meters
>
>Five times

37. Rope Work

>Twenty burpees
>
>Jump rope three minutes
>
>Five times

Alternatively, do twenty burpees and then jump rope for the remainder of the three minutes. Go directly into another three minutes of twenty burpees and jump roping. Do this for fifteen minutes.

38. World Tour

>Twenty burpees forward jump
>
>Bear crawl 150 feet (three times fifty feet for a small space)
>
>Frog squat jump fifty feet
>
>Five times

39. Lungs and Legs

>Twenty-five burpees
>
>Twenty-five barbell squats one hundred pounds/sixty-five pounds
>
>Twenty-five burpees
>
>Run a half mile
>
>Two times

40. The Nikki

Brutal!

>Ten burpees
>
>Ten slams
>
>Ten donkey kicks
>
>Five wall walks
>
>Ten times

This one will kick your ass.

41. Ross 500

>One hundred burpees
>
>One hundred rows
>
>One hundred squats

One hundred sit-ups

One hundred slams

Start with burpees, then do the rest in whichever order you want.

42. Dice Burpees

Get a pair of dice. Set a timer for four eight-minute rounds. The rounds will not have rests between them.

You will roll the dice, and the combined number will tell you what exercise you are doing (from the list below). For example, roll a "two," and you are doing ten inchworms.

After each exercise, complete ten burpees. Then roll again. Do your exercise and then complete ten burpees. Every time you roll, you do an exercise and then complete ten burpees! (Yes, this is an enormous number of burpees. If it's too much for you right now, cut the burpees to five reps.)

Do this for all four eight-minute rounds, but at the end of every eight minutes, you stop and run around the block (about a quarter mile, or two to three minutes). Start the eight-minute timer again before you run so that when you get back, you have about five minutes left in the eight-minute round. Then go back to the dice. Total workout is thirty-two minutes.

Exercises:

Two = ten inchworms

Three = fifteen diamond push-ups

Four = twenty frog squats

Five = twenty jump lunges

Six = forty mountain climbers

Seven = fifteen knee tucks

Eight = twenty squat thrusts

Nine = twenty-five squats

Ten = twenty lateral jumps

Eleven = twenty V-ups

Twelve = fifteen rows

43. Dice Burpees without Run

Just do dice burpees (see workout 42 above). Roll for the exercise and then do ten burpees.

Do this ten times until you hit one hundred burpees.

44. Jack

Ten burpees

Ten lunges

Ten squats

Twenty jumping jacks

Do this every two minutes for twenty minutes. Brutal!

45. Sit-ups Are Your Rest

Forty burpees, fifteen sit-ups

Thirty burpees, fifteen sit-ups

Twenty burpees, fifteen sit-ups

Ten burpees, fifteen sit-ups

46. Straight!

Talk about breathing fire. Do the burpees slower but do one hundred straight. To keep track, do a burpee and then say the number: "One." Then do another...just keep going, and don't stop until you reach one hundred.

47. Deck of Cards

Get a deck of cards. Each suit represents an exercise. Turn the cards over, and do the number of reps of the corresponding exercise.

Clubs = lunges

Diamonds = jumping jacks

Hearts = burpees

Spades = sit-ups

For cards valued at two though ten, do that many reps. Example: a six of hearts means six burpees.

J, Q, K = ten reps

A = sixteen reps

You will get one hundred of each exercise if you go through the entire deck (fifty-two cards).

48. Deck of Cards—Burpees Only

Flip the cards and do the corresponding number of burpees for the value of the card. For this workout, all face cards are ten and aces are eleven.

Do this until you get to one hundred burpees. Suit doesn't matter on this workout.

49. Penalty Burpees with Jump Rope

Begin by jumping rope. Every time you mess up, do ten burpees. Continue this until you hit one hundred burpees.

50. One Minute

Do burpees for one minute

Take one a one-minute rest

Repeat until you hit one hundred burpees.

51. Four minutes

Do burpees for four minutes (this is rough!)

Take a three-minute break

Repeat until you hit one hundred burpees.

52. Walk the Dog

Start by doing twenty burpees on your driveway or in your home. Then walk your dog. Every third house, do ten burpees!

53. Conditioning One Hundred

Bear crawl fifty feet down

Frog squat fifty feet back

Sprint down fifty feet and back

Do twenty burpees

Five times

54. Sean

Ten burpees

Ten slams

Ten rows

Ten SDBs (burpees with knee tucks)

Five times

55. Burpee Number[†]

Ten minutes of burpee number (ten one-minute rounds)

Run one mile

Finish with any burpees left

56. The Hills Are Alive

Ten burpees

Run up hill and walk down.

Ten V-ups

Fifty mountain climbers

Ten times

Tough!

[†] Burpee number is the number of burpees you can do in thirty seconds. Mine is ten, so I hit ten burpees every minute for ten minutes. Once I've done ten burpees, I rest for the remainder of the minute.

57. Calisthenics Are Easy

   Twenty-five burpees

   One hundred jumping jacks

   Twenty-five burpees

   One hundred mountain climbers

   Two times

58. Basic Tens

   Ten jump lunges

   Ten jump squats

   Ten rows

   Ten push-ups

   Ten burpees

   Ten times

This one might kill you!

59. A Buck and a Quarter

   One hundred jump rope turns

   Twenty-five burpees

   Four times

60. Quicksand

   (Ten dumbbell burpees) × ten

61. Scramble

   Ten lateral jump burpees

   Sprint down fifty feet

   Bear crawl back fifty feet

   Ten SDBs (burpees with knee tucks)

   Bear crawl backward down fifty feet

   Sprint back

   Five times

Whew!

62. Farm Hand

   Twenty burpees

   Farmer walk down fifty feet and back

   Ten slams

   Ten renegade rows

   Twenty burpees

   Two times

   Then finish with twenty slam burpees (medicine ball slam and burpee)

63. Fifty/Fifty and Some Change
>   Fifty burpees
>   Twenty donkey kicks
>   Twenty sit-outs
>   Twenty push-ups
>   Twenty rows or pull-ups
>   Run a half mile
>   Finish with fifty burpees

64. Slurpee on the Rocks
>   Twenty-five slams
>   Twenty-five burpees
>   Four times

65. Walk the Plank
>   Ten burpees
>   One minute of planks
>   Ten times

66. Run the Plank
>   Twenty burpees
>   One minute of planks
>   Five times

67. Ascending Ladder
>   Five burpees
>   Ten burpees
>   Fifteen burpees
>   Twenty burpees
>   Two times

>Rest as needed in between sets.

68. Deck of Cards: Full Workout II
>   Clubs = sit-outs
>   Diamonds = rows
>   Hearts = burpees
>   Spades = squats
>   Reps are value of card for number cards. Face cards are ten; aces are eleven.
>   End with five burpees.

69. Hard Body

> Ten dumbbell shoulder presses
>
> Ten curls
>
> Ten upright rows
>
> Ten squat thrusts
>
> Ten push-ups
>
> Ten V-ups
>
> Twenty-five burpees
>
> Four times

70. Back and Forth

> Twenty-five burpees forward jump (burpee and then broad jump forward)
>
> Backward bear crawl back to start
>
> Twenty-five burpees forward jump
>
> Crab walk back to start
>
> Twenty-five burpees forward jump
>
> Alligator crawl back (yes, brutal)
>
> Twenty-five burpees forward jump
>
> Bear crawl back to start

71. Sandbag's Your Buddy

> Ten sandbag shoulder burpees (do a burpee and then shoulder a sandbag)
>
> Ten sandbag Zercher squats (hold the sandbag in your arms)
>
> Ten burpee lateral sandbag jumps (lay the sandbag down, do a burpee on one side of it, jump over the sandbag, and do another burpee)
>
> Ten sandbag Zercher squats
>
> Ten sandbag clean and press
>
> Five times

Tough stuff!

72. Mix It Up

> Ten burpees lateral jump left
>
> Ten burpees lateral jump right
>
> Ten SDBs (burpees with knee tucks)
>
> Ten burpees feet wide
>
> Ten burpees feet close together
>
> Two times

73. Ten Burpee Ten Run

Ten burpees

Ten sprints (fifty feet)

Ten times

74. Fun Bucket

Cut up slips of paper. Write the numbers two, four, six, eight, ten, twelve, fifteen, and twenty-five on different slips.

Put them in a shoebox or a bucket and mix them up. Draw a slip of paper and do the number of reps it says. Do this until you get to one hundred. Try to do them without stopping during the set. If your last slip puts you over one hundred, try to do the number on the slip anyway.

75. Roll for Burpees

Roll two dice and do the number of reps. Repeat until you get to one hundred.

76. Five × Twenty

Do five burpees

Take three to five big breaths

Repeat for twenty sets

77. One Hundred Around-the-World Burpees

Burpee with a jump forward

Burpee with a jump right

Burpee with a jump back

Burpee with a jump left (you just made a square)

Twenty-five times

78. Arms and Burpees

Ten curls

Ten tricep overhead presses

Ten burpees

Ten times

79. The Mountain

One hundred burpees

Two hundred abs (fifty sit-ups, fifty reverse crunches, fifty V-ups, fifty leg raises)

Three hundred squats

Four hundred mountain climbers

This is a mountain of misery! (The good kind!)

80. **The Beast**
> One hundred burpees
> Two hundred push-ups
> Three hundred crunches
> Four hundred squats

This is a *beast*!

81. **Fatigue**
> Ten burpees
> Sprint four times (down and back twice) thirty to fifty yards
> Ten burpees
> Walk down and back to recover
> Five times

82. **Triple Threat**
> Ten burpees
> Ten squats
> Ten sit-ups
> Ten times

83. **Just Breathe**
> Ten burpees
> Ten slams
> Bear crawl down fifty feet and back
> Ten SDBs (burpees with knee tucks)
> Five times

Smoker!

84. **Cardio Burpees**
> Treadmill run or bike two minutes
> Fifteen burpees

Repeat until you reach one hundred.

85. **Squat Burpees**
> Ten barbell squats
> Ten burpees
> Ten times

86. **One hundred-Burpee Mile**
> Twenty-five burpees
> Immediately run a mile, but stop three times along the way, doing twenty-five burpees each time

87. **Fifty-Burpee Miles**

> Twenty burpees
>
> Immediately run a mile
>
> Stop three times along the way, doing ten burpees each time
>
> Repeat

88. **Six-Pack**

> Twenty-five burpees
>
> Run a quarter mile
>
> Twenty-five sit-ups
>
> One minute of planks
>
> Four times

89. **Egyptian Sets**

> Two × five burpees
>
> Two × ten burpees
>
> Two × twenty burpees
>
> Two × ten burpees
>
> Two × five burpees

90. **The Climb**

> Two × five burpees
>
> Two × ten burpees
>
> Two × twenty burpees
>
> One × thirty burpees (do these straight at the end!)

91. **Serious Legs**

> Twenty-five burpees
>
> Twenty-five reverse squats
>
> Twenty-five lunges
>
> Twenty-five high knees
>
> Twenty-five boot strappers
>
> Four times

92. **Barbell Complex and Burpees**

> Six dead lifts
>
> Six front squats
>
> Six shoulder presses
>
> Six back squats
>
> Six upright rows
>
> Six curls
>
> Twenty burpees

Five times

Use a light weight. The weight should be light enough to do your weakest exercise without changing the weights. The idea is to do all six exercises for six reps without taking a break. Rest after you complete the complex before the burpees. It is brutal—strength *and* cardio!

93. The List

Set a timer for forty-five minutes. Go down the list and complete as much as you can!

> One hundred crunches
>
> Thirty-five V-ups
>
> Twenty leg raises
>
> One hundred push-ups
>
> One hundred squats
>
> Five hundred mountain climbers (that's right—it may take eight to ten minutes)
>
> Fifty burpees
>
> Run two times around the block (or approximately four to five minutes)
>
> Twenty-five burpees
>
> Two minutes of plank
>
> Fifty dumbbell swings
>
> One hundred jumping jacks
>
> Twenty-five burpees
>
> Forty sit-ups
>
> Fifty push jacks
>
> Fifty sit-outs

If time runs out, add on how many burpees you need to reach one hundred. If you finish early, you are done! Go get it! You will be surprised at how much you can do!

94. Two-Mile Shit Sandwich

> Run one mile
>
> One hundred burpees
>
> Run one mile

95. Twenty Minutes

> One minute of burpees
>
> One minute of dumbbell high knees (or jumping jacks if no dumbbells)
>
> Ten times

If you still have burpees left, pound them out at the end. Brutal!

96. Full-Body Minutes

> One minute of burpees
>
> One minute of sit-ups
>
> One minute of burpees
>
> One minute of squats
>
> One minute of burpees
>
> One minute of jumping jacks

Keep repeating this until you reach one hundred burpees!

97. Jumpees Mile Sandwich

> (Long jump one hundred feet and do twenty-five burpees) × two
>
> Run one mile
>
> (Long jump one hundred feet and do twenty-five burpees) × two

98. Slow and Steady

> Five burpees every minute for twenty minutes

99. Sports or TV Burpees

> Every commercial break, get up and do burpees until you reach one hundred.

100. SDBs

> One hundred SDBs (burpees with knee tucks)

Do them any way you can (ten × ten, five × twenty, etc.)

101. Burps and Jacks

> Ten burpees
>
> Forty jumping jacks
>
> Ten times

102. Suicide Burpees

> One minute of burpees
>
> One minute suicide run
>
> One minute of burpees
>
> Rest

Repeat this as many times as you need to reach one hundred burpees. Keep track on paper for this one, because it's easy to get confused.

103. Basics Plus Fifty-Burpee Mile

> Ten burpees
>
> Ten lunges
>
> Ten push-ups

Ten squats
Five times
And then do a fifty-burpee mile!

There were three extra workouts! We always try to overdeliver (and so should you)! A baker's dozen makes for good business.

These workouts kick ass. We know because we've done them—and so have our peeps.

Now remember, watching someone score a touchdown and actually scoring a touchdown yourself produce two very different experiences. It's time for you to score a few workout "touchdowns." It's time to get in the game. Don't just read the workouts. Do one.

Pick one and do it. Pick one that scares you, and finish it! No more BS. You will feel like Rocky Balboa with your arms raised at the end! "Yoooo, Adrian! I did it!"

Have fun. (Cue sinister, evil laugh.)

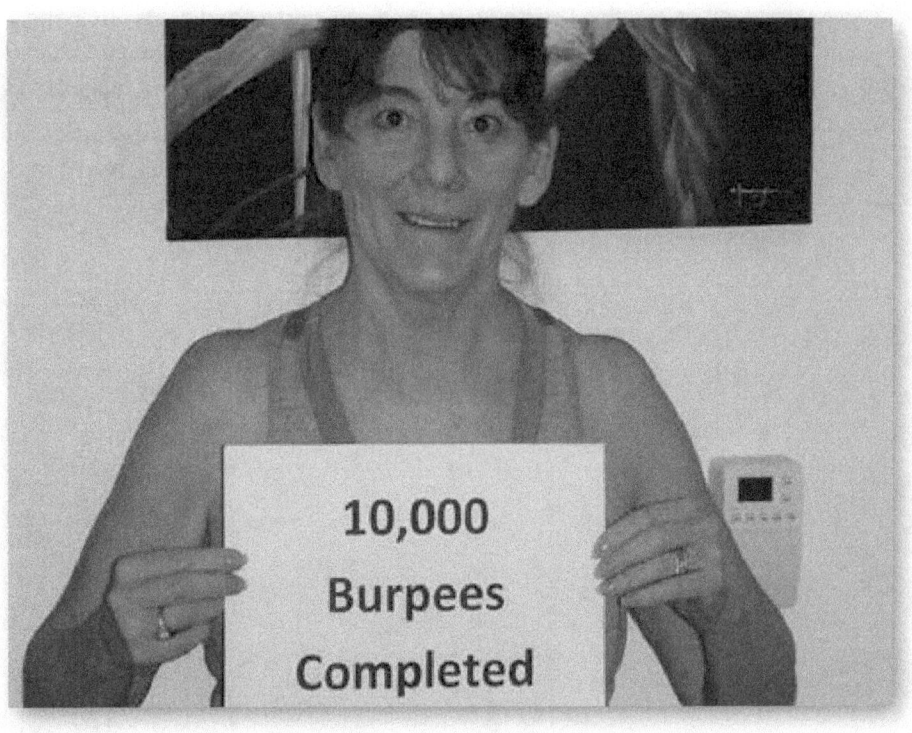

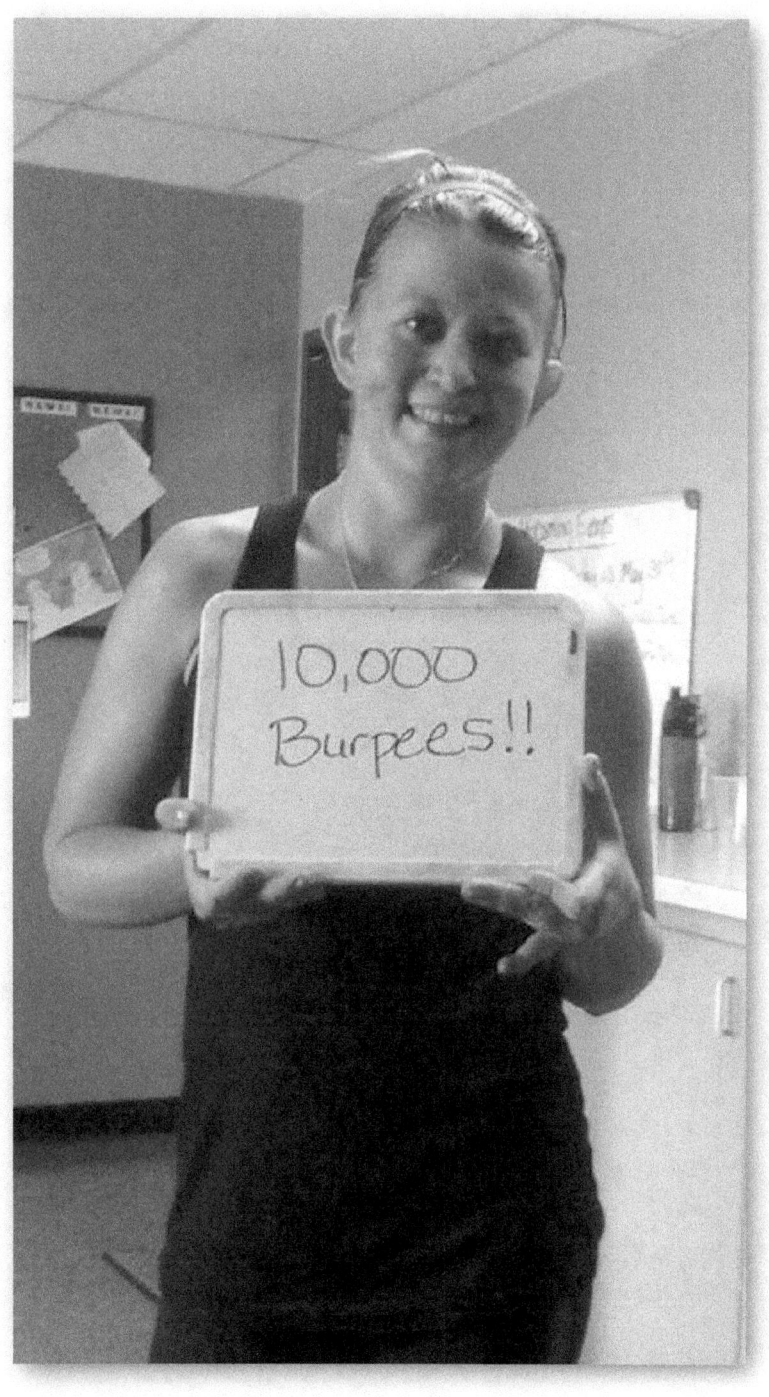

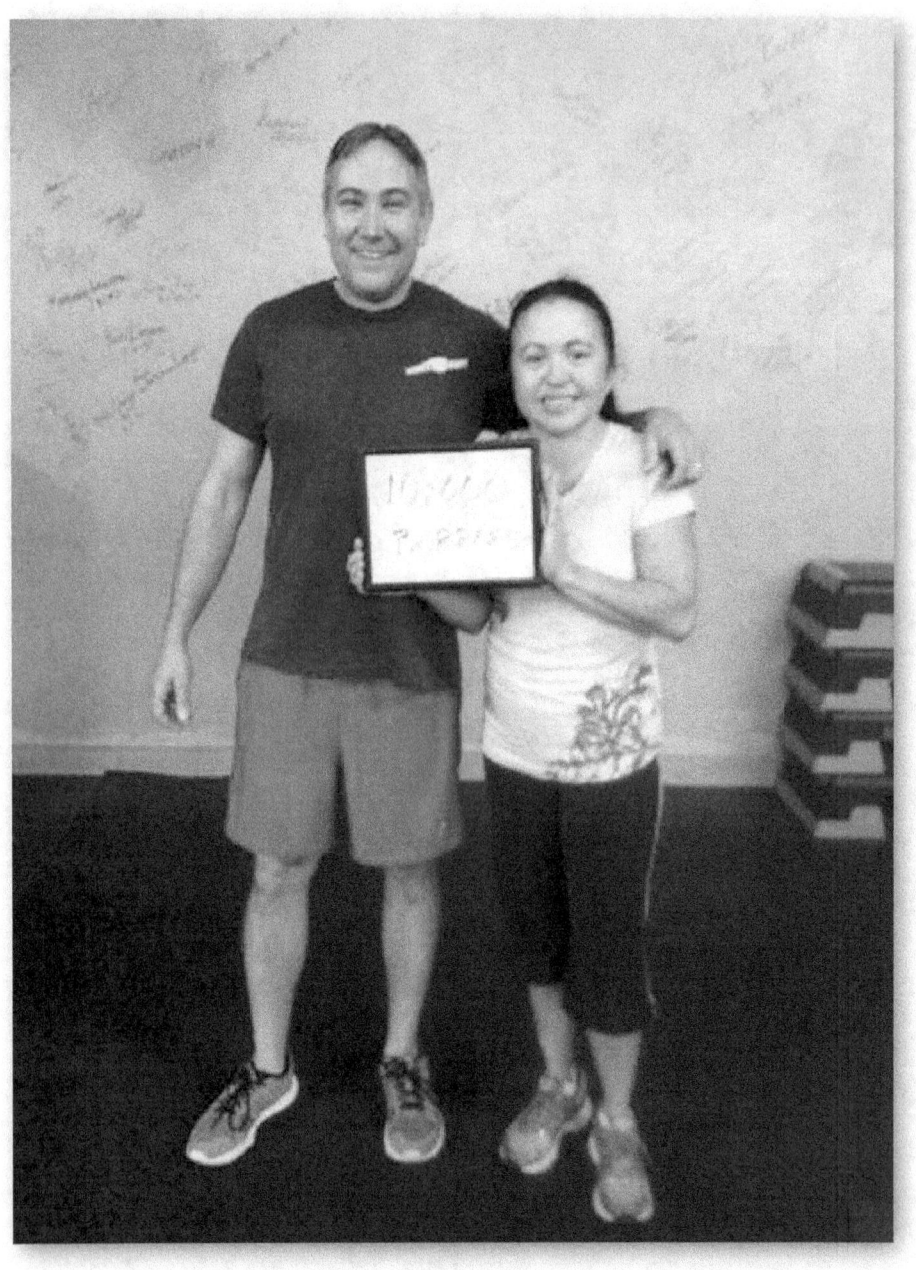

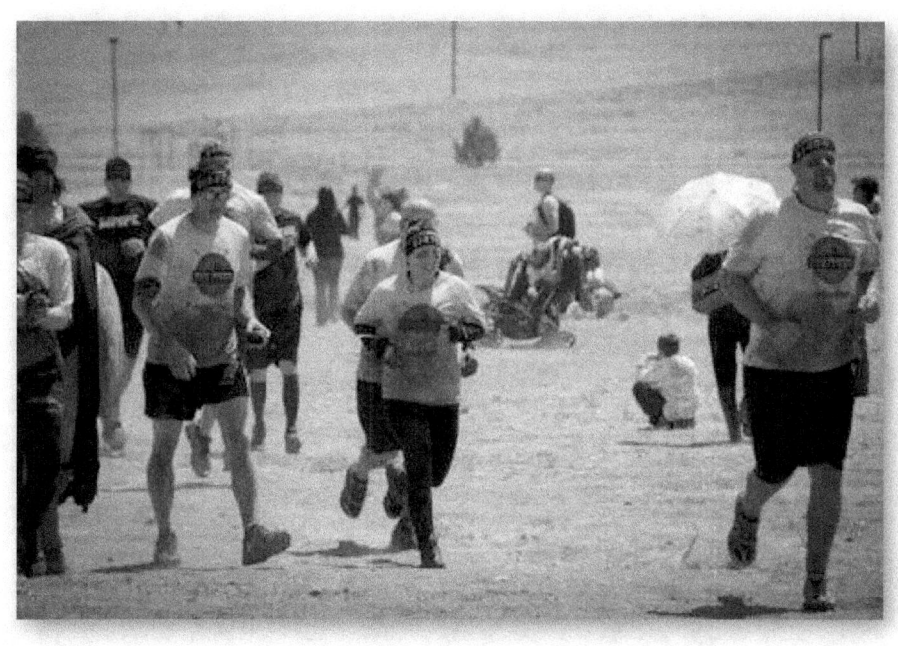

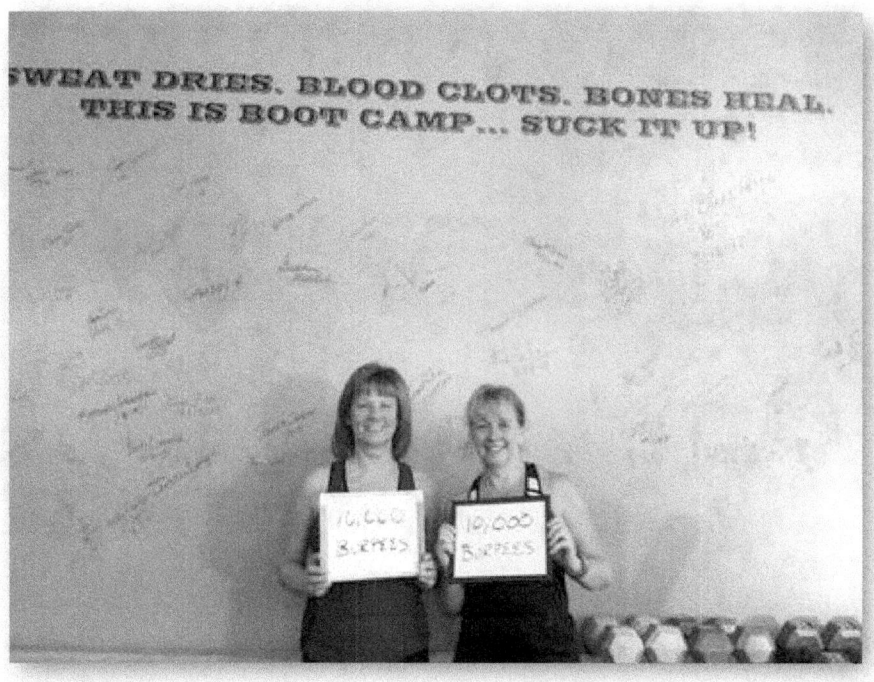

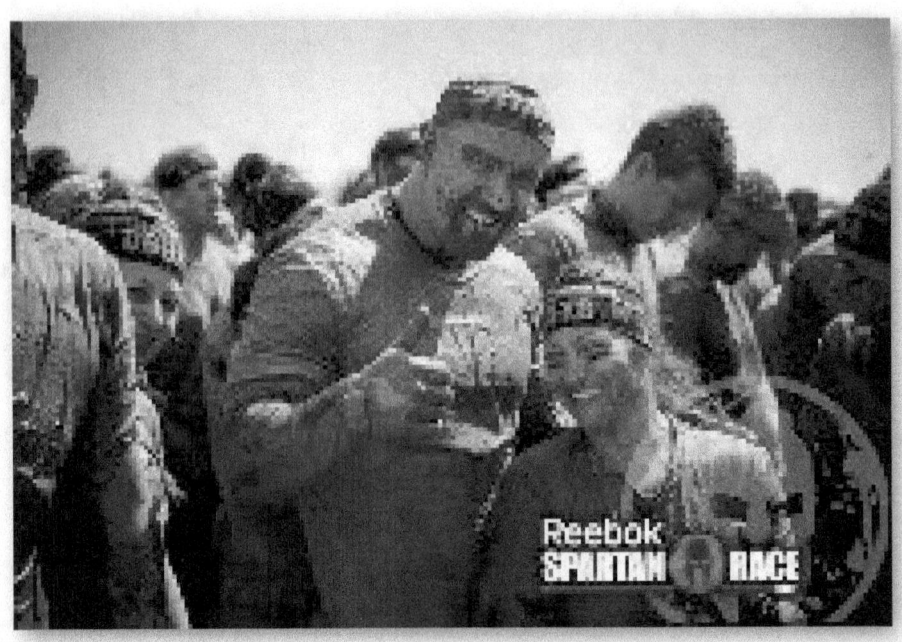

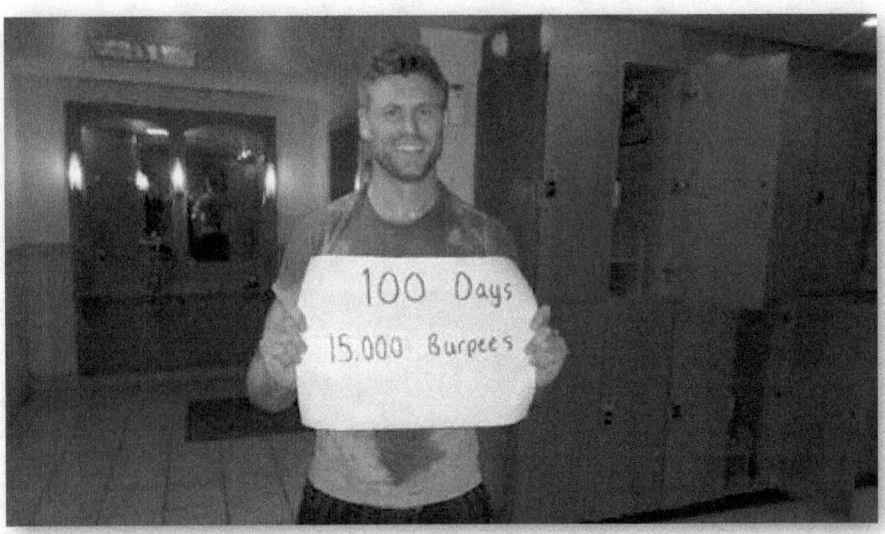

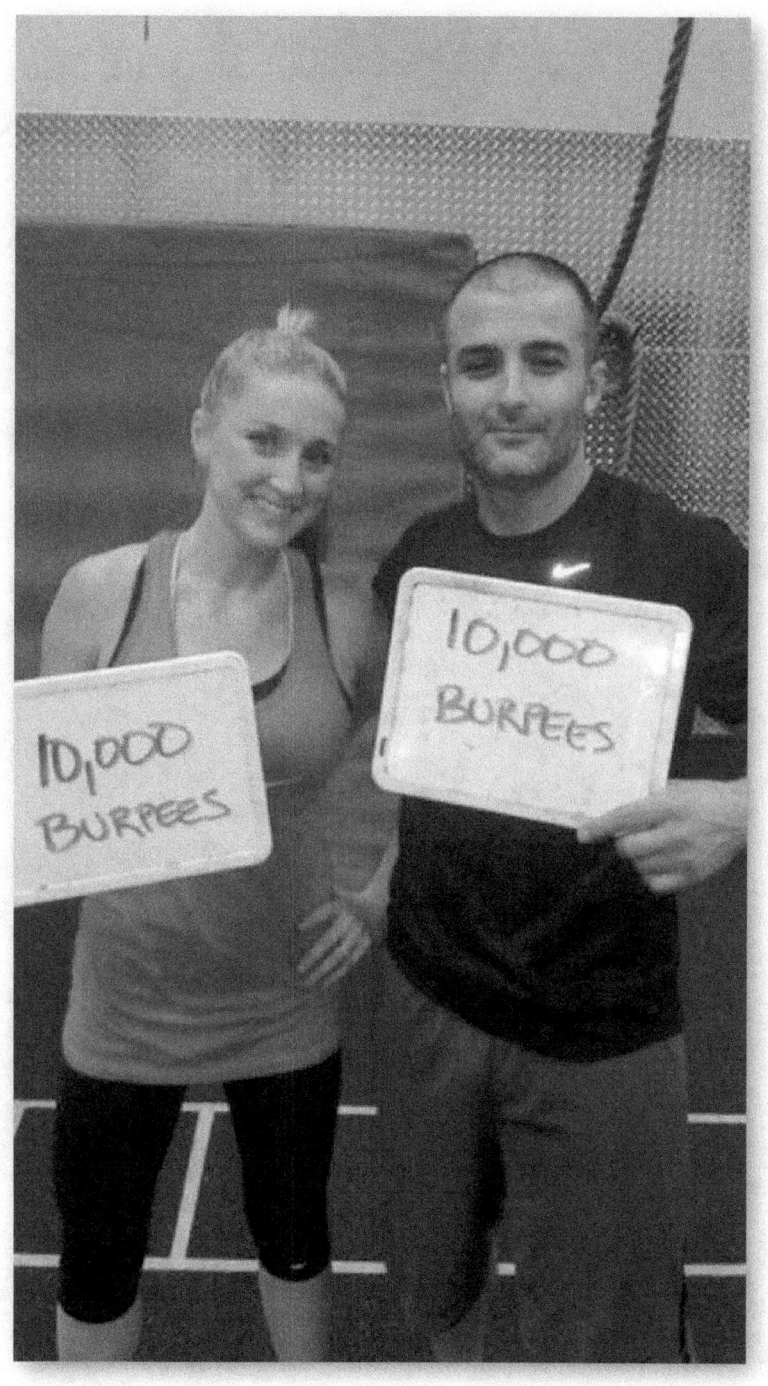

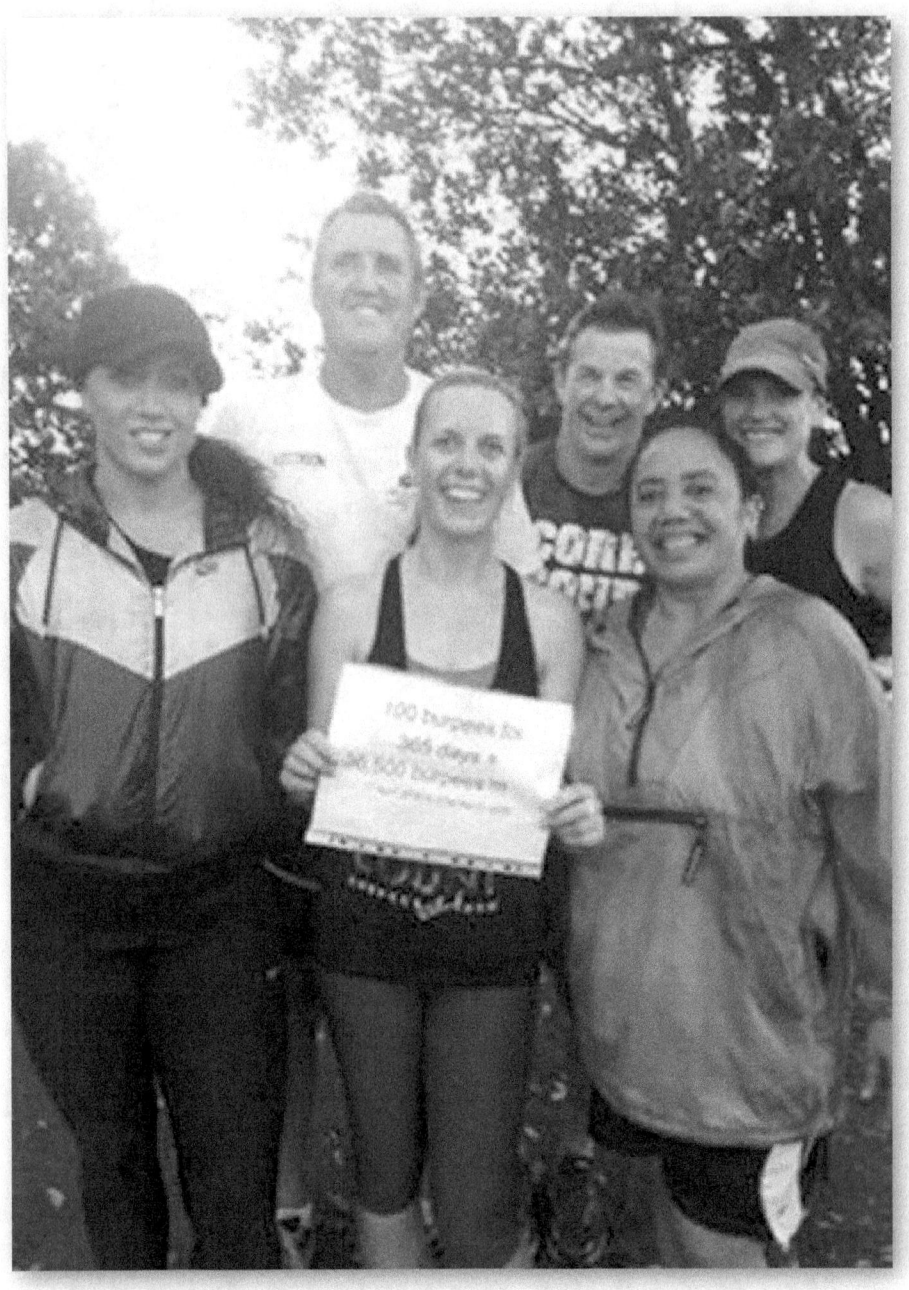

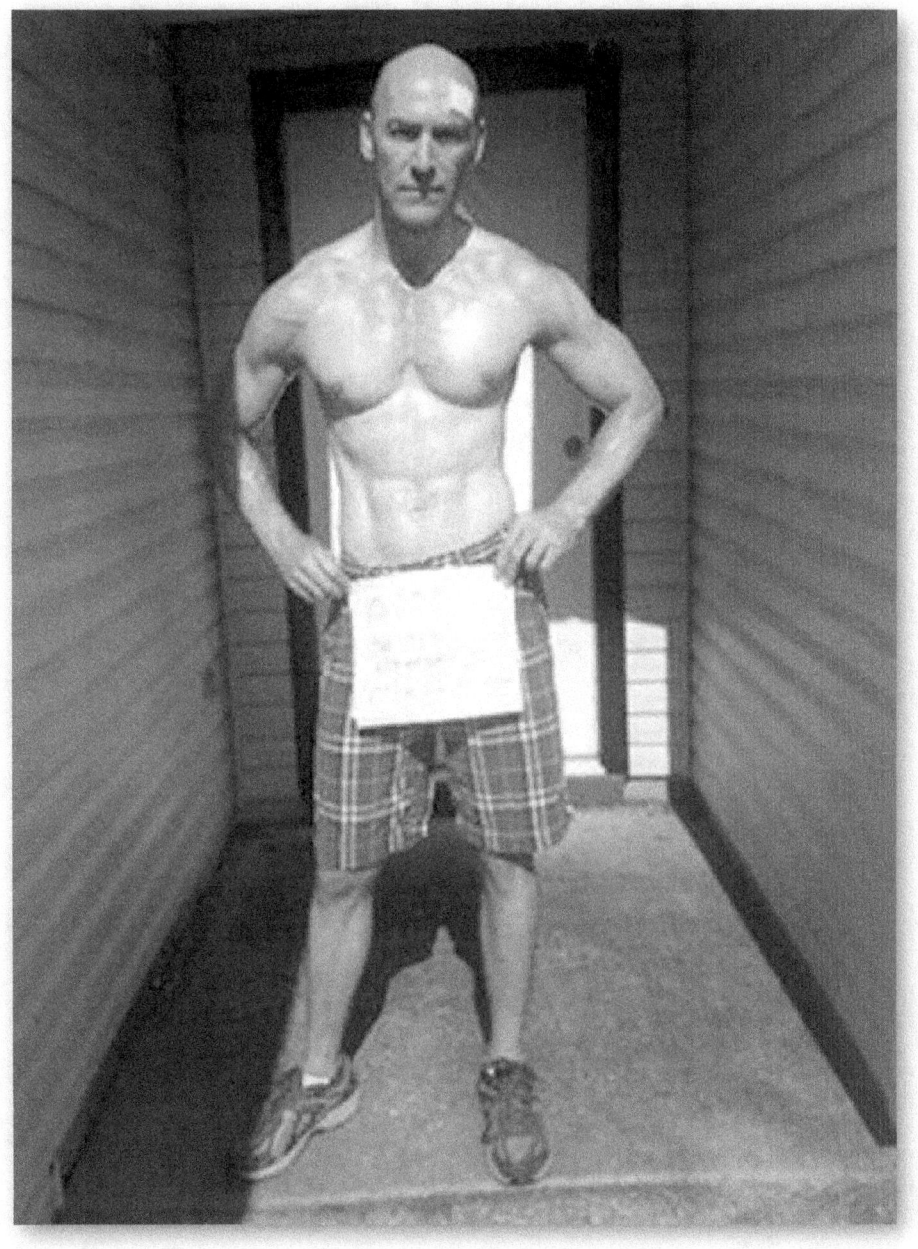

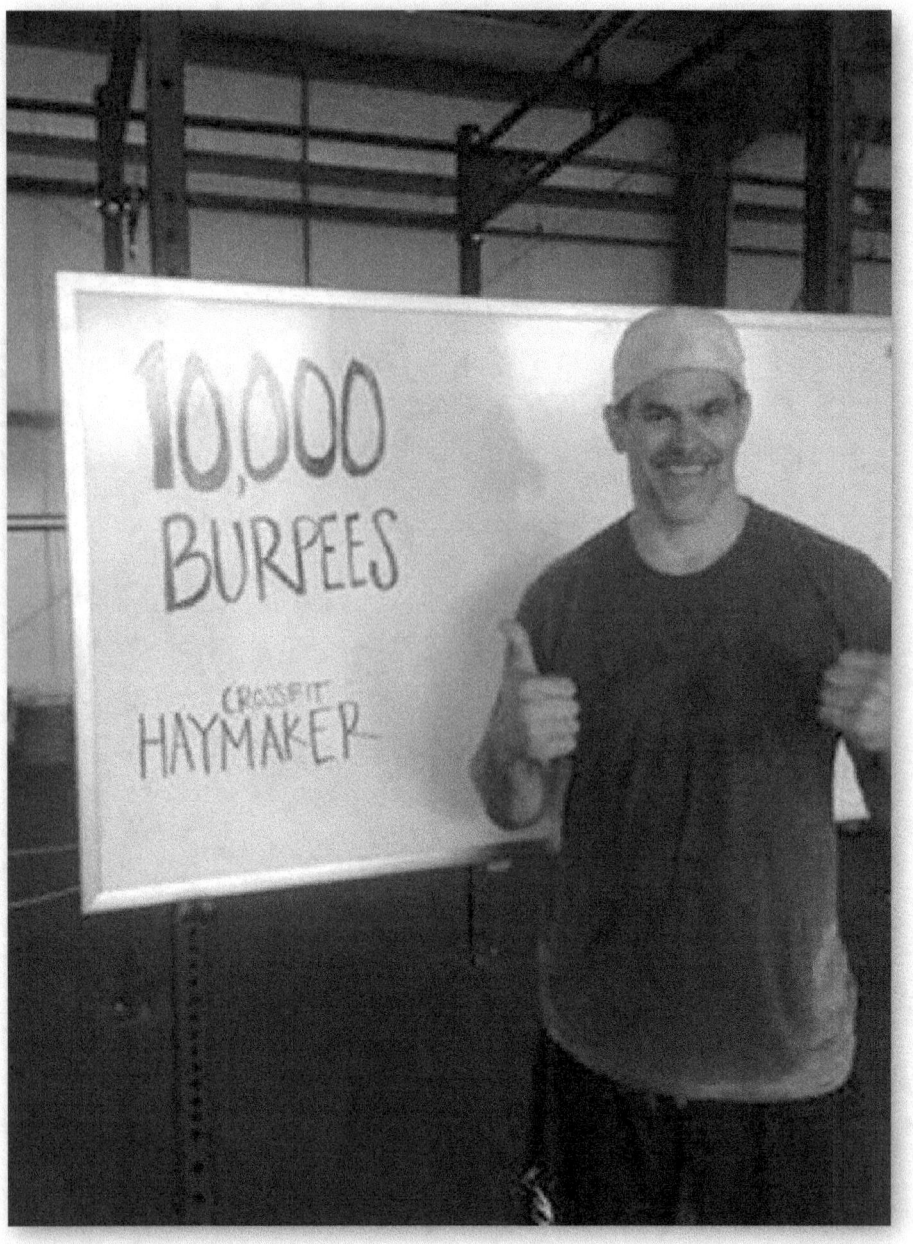

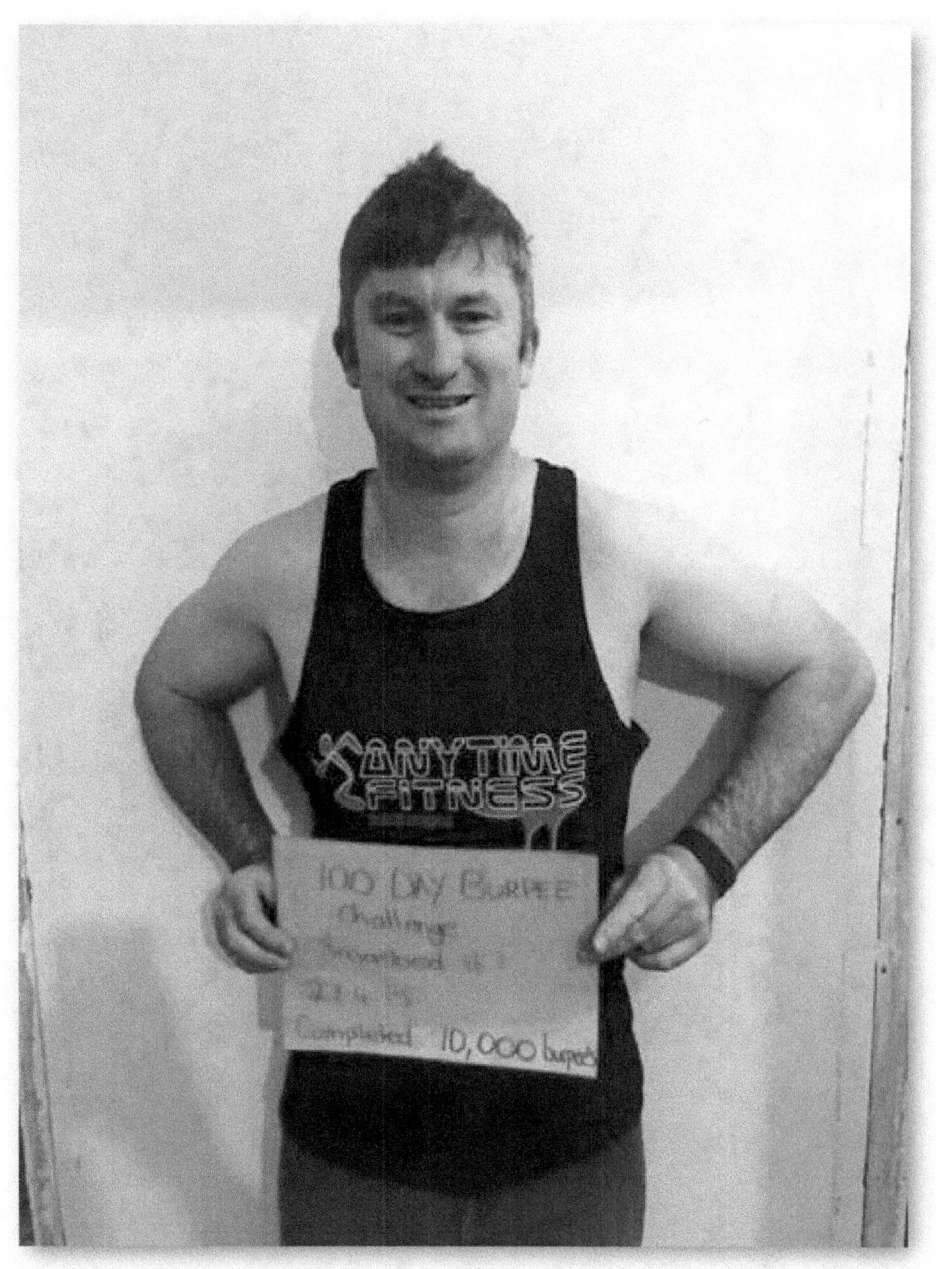

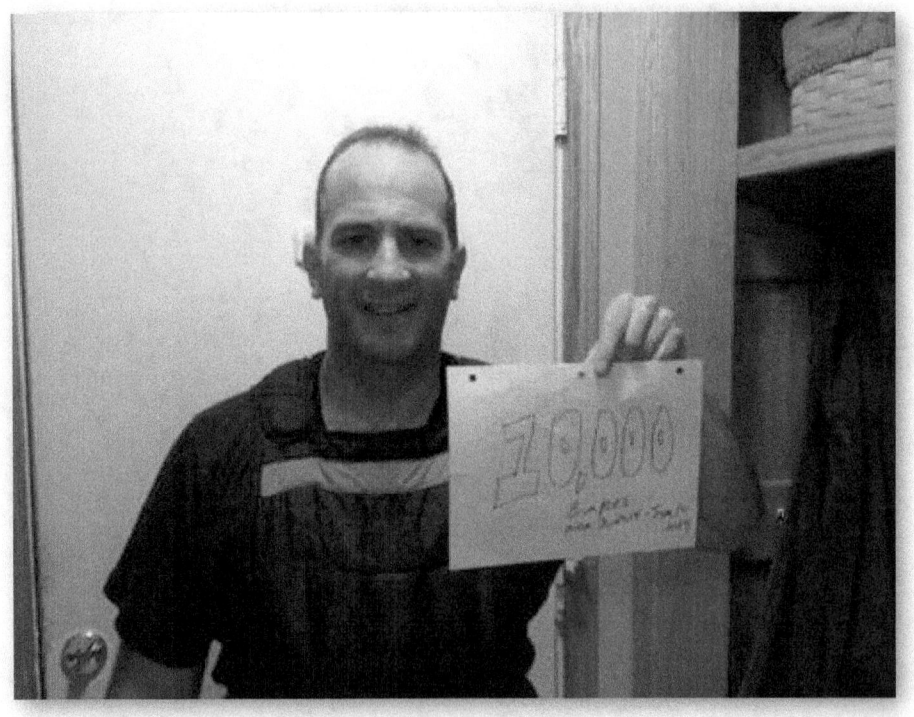

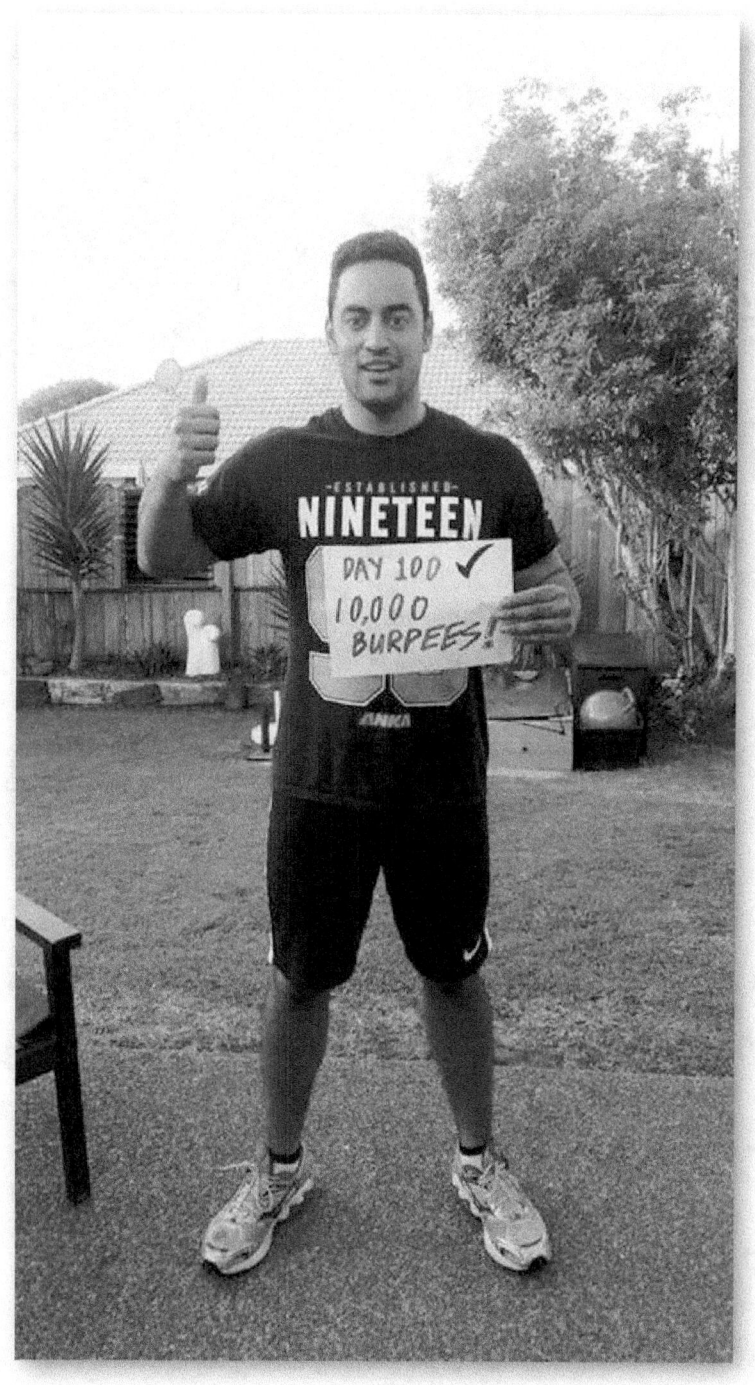

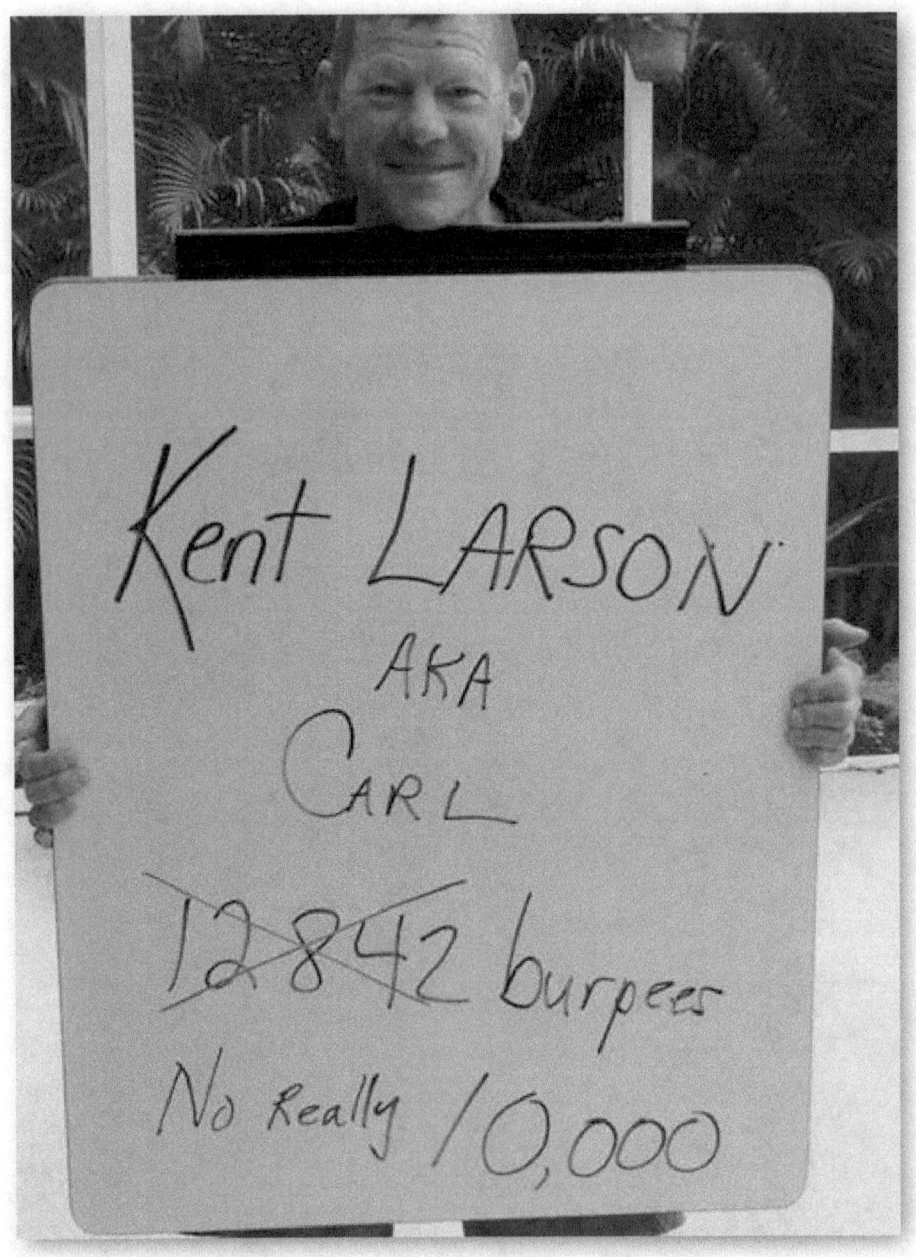

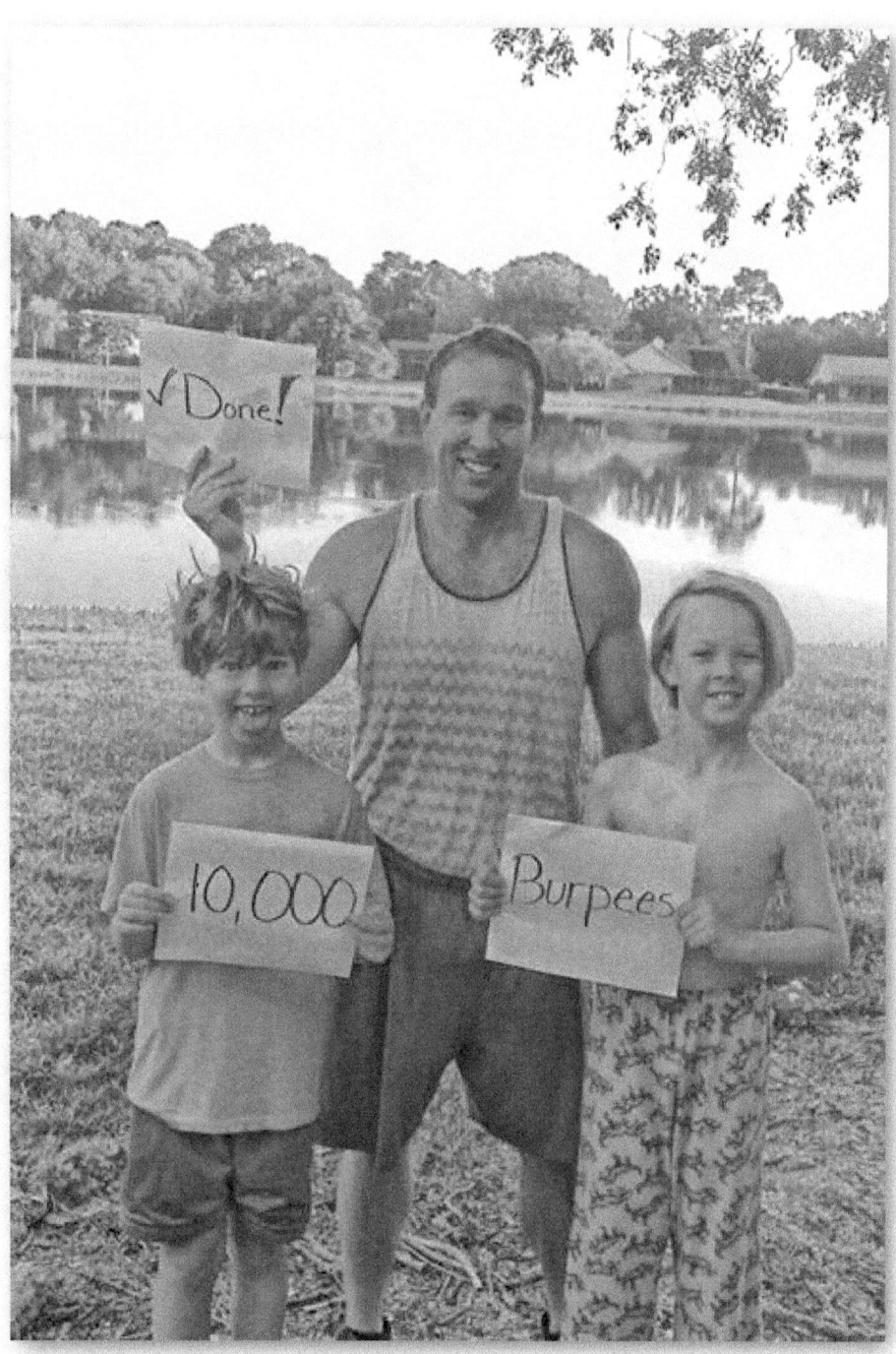

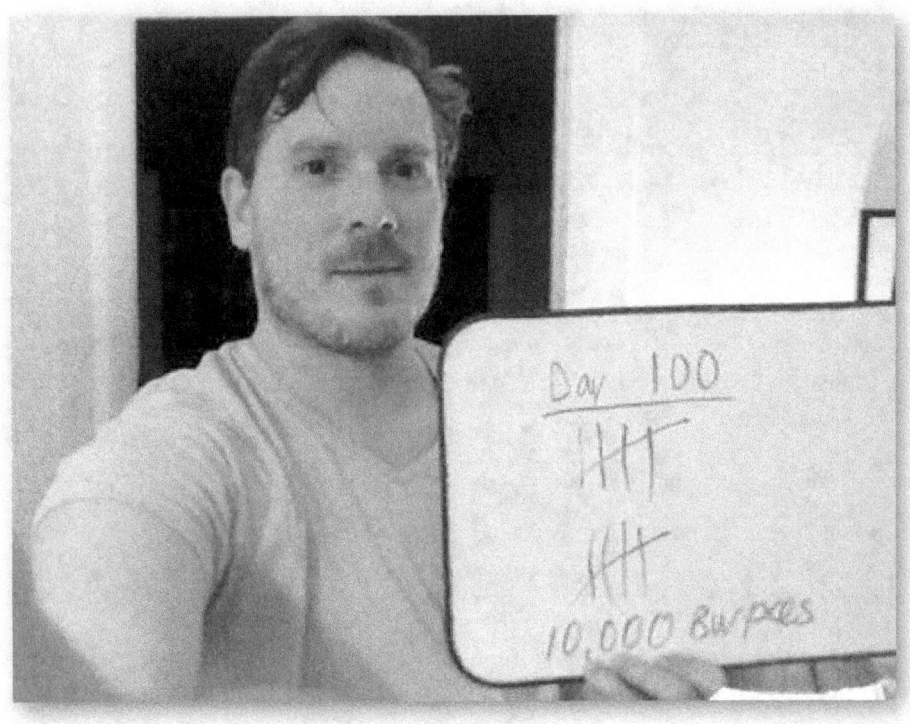

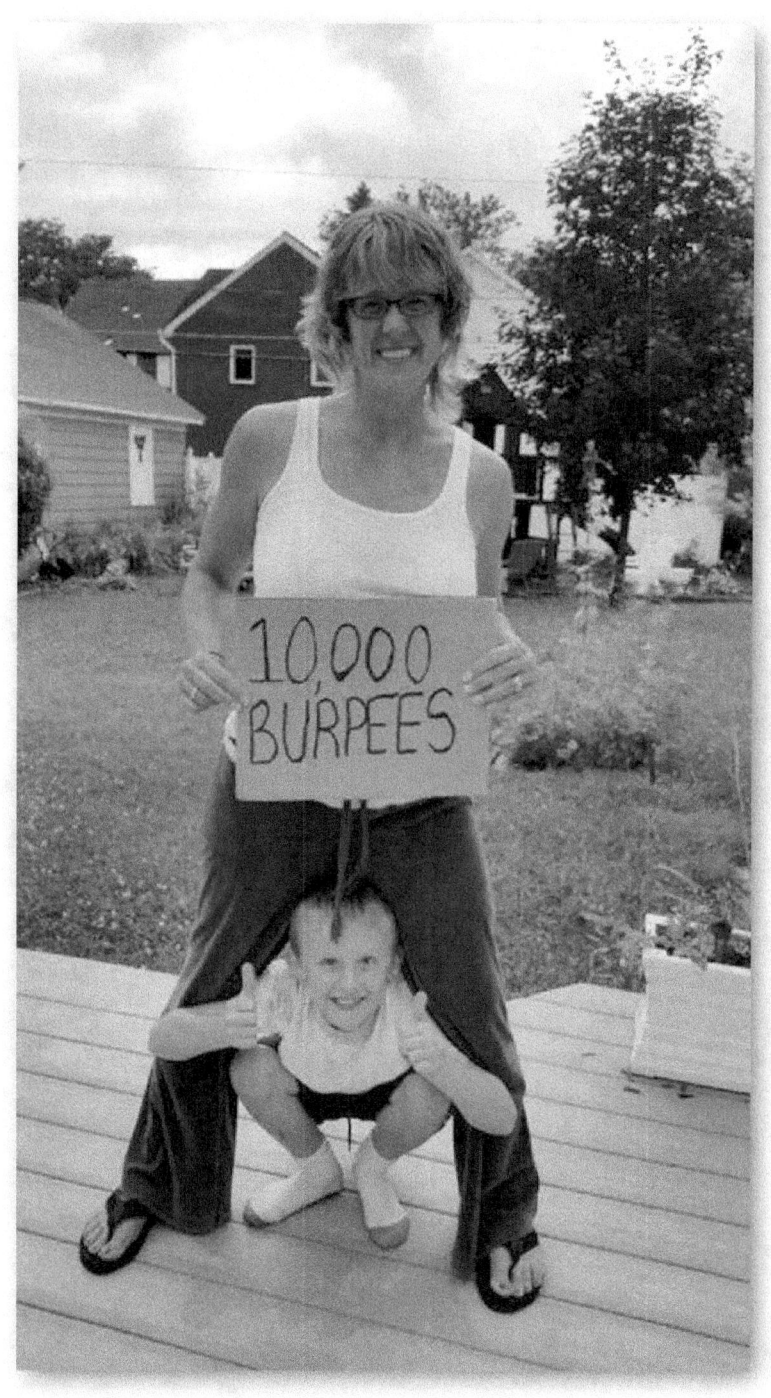

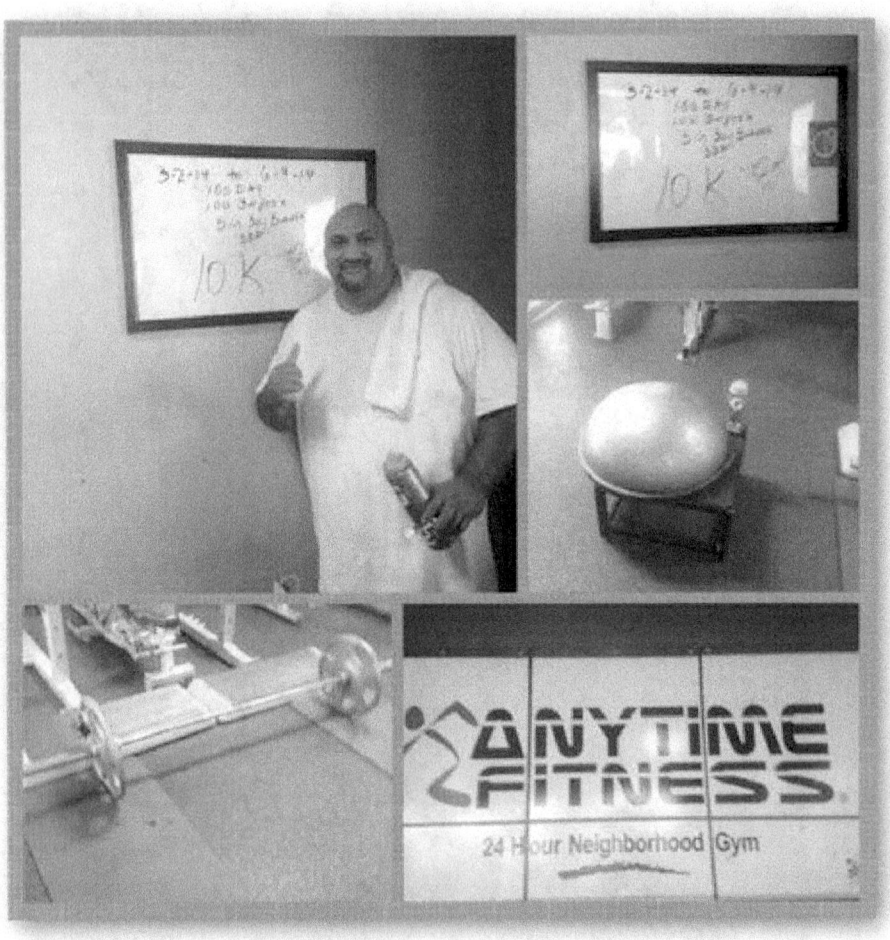

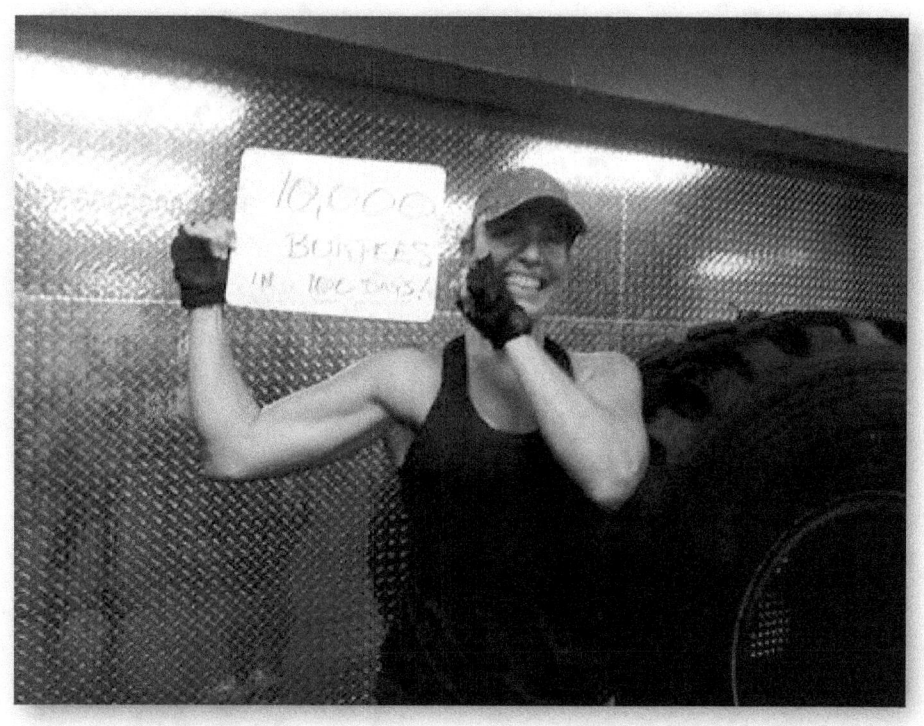

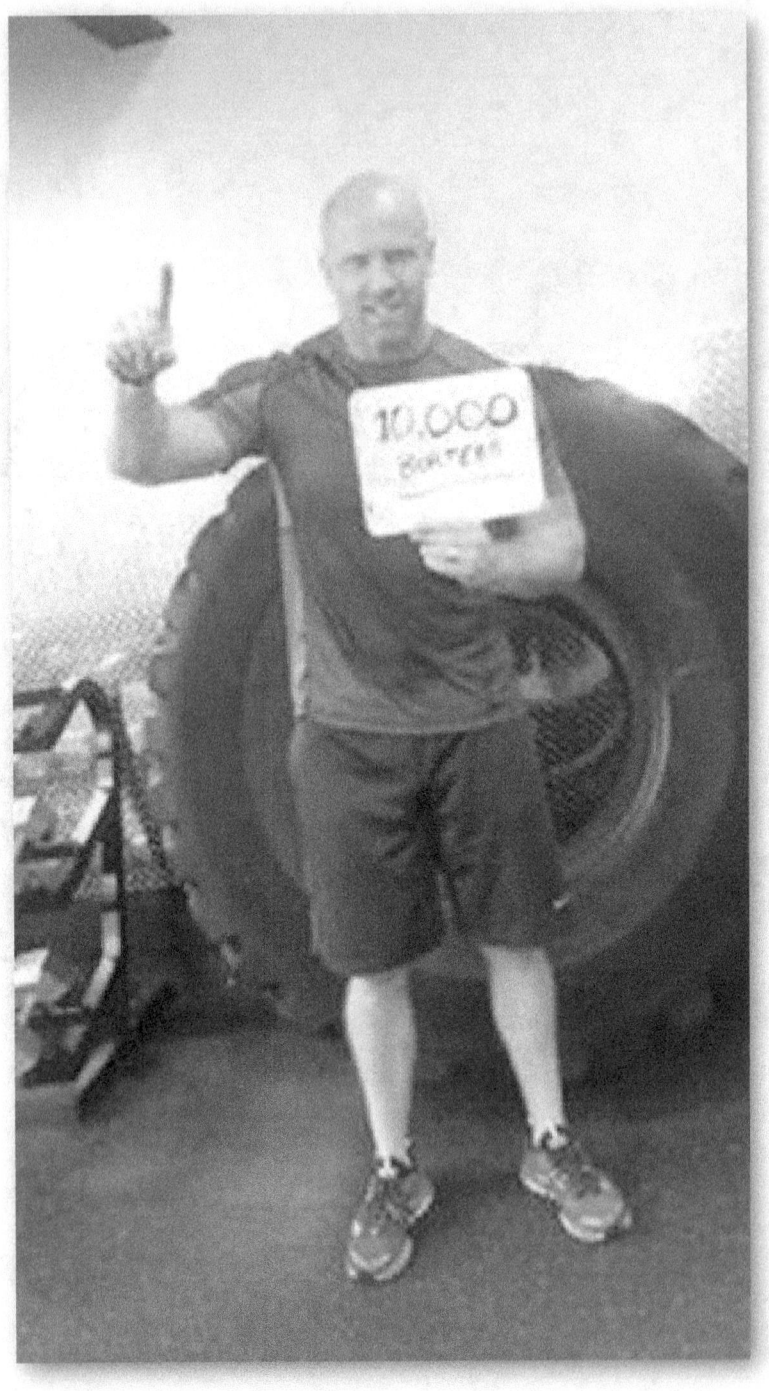

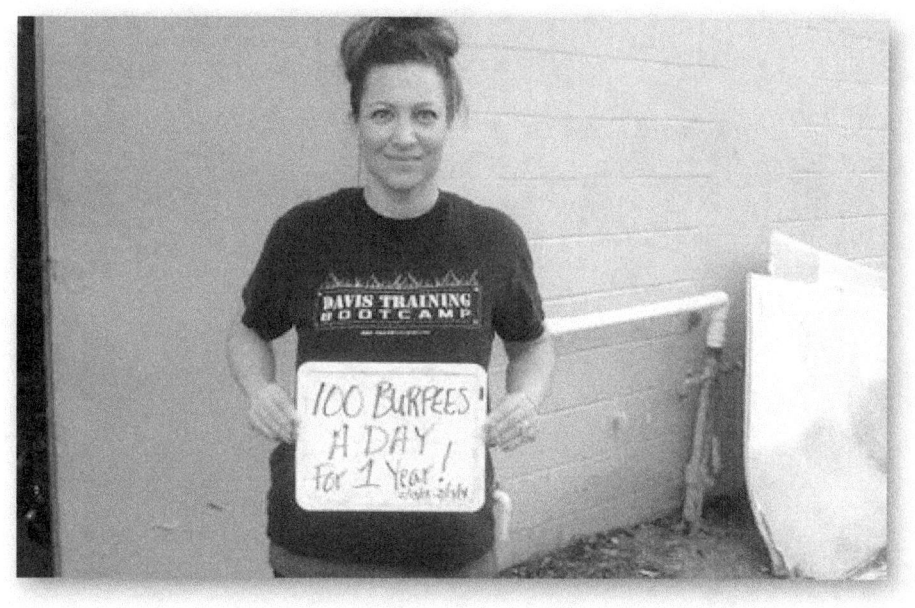

www.ingramcontent.com/pod-product-compliance
Lightning Source LLC
Chambersburg PA
CBHW060432290526
45791CB00002B/930